WRITING SKILLS FOR NURSING AND MIDWIFERY STUDENTS

SAGE has been part of the global academic community since 1965, supporting high quality research and learning that transforms society and our understanding of individuals, groups and cultures. SAGE is the independent, innovative, natural home for authors, editors and societies who share our commitment and passion for the social sciences.

Find out more at: **www.sagepublications.com**

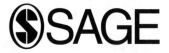

WRITING SKILLS FOR NURSING AND MIDWIFERY STUDENTS

DENA BAIN TAYLOR
↗

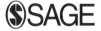

Los Angeles | London | New Delhi
Singapore | Washington DC

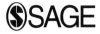

Los Angeles | London | New Delhi
Singapore | Washington DC

SAGE Publications Ltd
1 Oliver's Yard
55 City Road
London EC1Y 1SP

SAGE Publications Inc.
2455 Teller Road
Thousand Oaks, California 91320

SAGE Publications India Pvt Ltd
B 1/I 1 Mohan Cooperative Industrial Area
Mathura Road
New Delhi 110 044

SAGE Publications Asia-Pacific Pte Ltd
3 Church Street
#10-04 Samsung Hub
Singapore 049483

© Dena Bain Taylor 2013

First published 2013

Library of Congress Control Number: 2012937600

British Library Cataloguing in Publication data

A catalogue record for this book is available from
the British Library

Editor: Susan Worsey
Assistant Editor: Emma Milman
Production editor: Katie Forsythe
Copyeditor: Rosemary Morlin
Proofreader: Kate Scott
Marketing manager: Tamara Navaratnam
Cover design: Wendy Scott
Typeset by: C&M Digitals (P) Ltd, Chennai, India
Printed by MPG Books Group, Bodmin, Cornwall

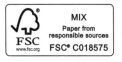

MIX
Paper from
responsible sources
FSC
www.fsc.org   FSC® C018575

ISBN 978-1-4462-0833-5
ISBN 978-1-4462-0834-2 (pbk)

TABLE OF CONTENTS

ABOUT THE AUTHOR

Dena Bain Taylor holds a PhD in English from the University of Toronto, Canada, where she has taught since 1985. As Director of the Health Sciences Writing Centre, she has 18 years of interdisciplinary experience teaching writing and critical skills across the full range of health professions, most notably with undergraduate and graduate students in the Lawrence S. Bloomberg Faculty of Nursing, Canada's largest school of Nursing. In 2012 she was awarded the University of Toronto's prestigious Joan E. Foley Award for Quality of Student Experience. Her academic publications include the *Young Learner's Illustrated English-Chinese Dictionary* (1994) and the online *Writing in the Health Sciences: A Comprehensive Guide* (2008). She lives in a small palace in the sky overlooking Lake Ontario.

ACKNOWLEDGMENTS

SAGE and the author would like to thank the following for the invaluable student essay examples included in the text.

Edwina Brako,
a student at the University of Toronto.

Jordan Chu,
a student at the University of Toronto.

Lisa Holland,
a student at the University of Glamorgan.

Laura Wright,
a student at the University of Glamorgan.

Kelly Crofts
a student at the University of Toronto.

Gemma Barnacle,
a student at the University of Chester.

Thanks is also due to:

Mark Broom, Senior Lecturer at the University of Glamorgan for his invaluable support in organising the student essay examples.

Jose Gibbs, Lecturer at Canterbury Christ Church University for her invaluable help in organising student essay examples.

Amanda Bennie, a student at Canterbury Christ Church University for her student essay example.

INTRODUCTION 1

CLEAR THINKING = CLEAR WRITING

Has this happened to you? You have a writing assignment due in two or three weeks, so, as a good time manager, you start working on it now. But you don't seem to get anywhere. You spend a great deal of time reading course materials and journal articles; you take notes; you write an outline; you struggle to come up with a first page; and in general feel frustrated that so much time has produced so little. Suddenly your deadline is upon you and in the last few days before the paper is due, the mental floodgates open and out pours the paper. Exhausted, you hand it in and wonder, why couldn't I have done this the first week and saved myself all that time and trouble?

The answer is that clear thinking takes time to develop, and only clear thinking leads to clear writing. Thinking and writing are what we call iterative processes, meaning that they develop each other in a back-and-forth process. In other words, writing is a form of thinking.

Tip: writing is a form of thinking

When you read and make notes, then go handle something else in your busy schedule, your mind continues to process what you've read. Even when you experience writer's block or you procrastinate – preferring to wash the car than to sit back down to write – your brain is still working. Bit by bit, your thoughts on your topic become more clear; one by one the right words to express those thoughts come to you. At a certain point, the results of that thinking process meet up with the impending deadline, and the paper gets written.

ABOUT THIS BOOK

Following the example of the Royal College of Nursing I use the word 'nursing' throughout to refer to the whole family of nursing, including midwifery and other allied health professions.

Worldwide, nursing is the largest of the health professions. To prepare students for today's complex health care environment, nursing and midwifery programs require students to engage in a wide variety of types of writing, from research papers and literature reviews, to clinical reports, to health promotion materials, to emails and online course discussions. As a student in a college or university program, you are learning to communicate in writing to a variety of potential career audiences that include – first and most important – your patients and the public, but also your colleagues, allied health professionals, administrators, agencies, the justice system and others. Like any professional skill, writing can be learned. Thus, the goal of this book is to show you how to write persuasively and correctly, both to support you in your courses and to prepare you for your professional careers.

This book aims to help you master the writing process and teach you the flexibility to tackle any form of communication your course instructors or your career ask of you. It approaches writing skills by focusing on both clear thinking (your ideas and the strategies for conveying them persuasively) and clear writing (the 'correct' way to write in nursing). The intention of the chapters in the first half is to establish a solid base of reading, writing, and critical argument skills. Although this book is intended for students at any level of study, if you are beginning your college or university program of study you will find Chapters 2 and 3 especially relevant. Chapter 2 presents practical strategies to manage your life and work to increase success and reduce stress. Chapter 3 sets out the fundamentals of the writing process and tips for navigating it successfully. Chapter 4 covers the foundational skills of writing clearly and persuasively. This section is not intended as a grammar text for students who are seeking extensive description of the general rules and conventions of English grammar and usage. Rather, it focuses on those rules and conventions as they relate to the health professions. Finally, Chapter 5 offers strategies for constructing a persuasive argument.

The second half of the book moves on to more advanced topics, beginning with how to use and acknowledge sources (Chapter 6). Chapter 7 covers the crucial skill of literature review, and Chapter 8, its companion, describes how to analyze and critically appraise the research literature. Chapter 9 moves away from academic writing to cover various forms of professional writing and communication. Chapter 10 addresses presentation skills, which are important in both the professional and academic worlds. To help you become a reflective practitioner, Chapter 11 offers a number of ways to engage in reflective writing. Finally, Chapter 12 consists of a set of sample student papers, to demonstrate some of the forms of writing you are likely to encounter in your course assignments.

A FEW ACKNOWLEDGMENTS

Finally, in many ways this book represents a sort of 'view from my desk'. Over the last 17 years, as director of the Health Sciences Writing Centre at the University of Toronto, Canada, I have worked one-on-one with thousands of students from across the full spectrum of the health professions, from the narrowly biomedical to the broadly sociocultural. They have enriched my understanding of the experience of learning to write, and knowing these students has enriched my personal life beyond words to express. It is to them that I owe my greatest thanks.

I'd also like to acknowledge the following colleagues at the University of Toronto who have kindly given me permission to adapt their instructional materials for this book: Dr Margaret Procter on plagiarism, Leora Freedman on writing a résumé, and Dr Nellie Perret for the glossary of 'Common Essay and Exam Directions'. I am grateful for the advice of other U of T colleagues on particular sections of the book: Dr Marius Locke on conciseness in scientific writing; Dr Lynda Mainwaring on research design; Dr Roxanne Power on professional and agency writing; Dr Timothy N Welsh on brain plasticity; and Debbie Green, Robarts Librarian, on types of literature. I also received very helpful advice from Alexandra Mayeski of Dykeman Dewhirst O'Brien Health Law, on witness statements; and Shannon Abbaterusso, RN, on clinical documentation. Finally, I owe a debt of gratitude to my family and friends for putting up with my writerly quirks and absences as I worked through this book.

ESSENTIAL MANAGEMENT AND STUDY SKILLS

2

THE VIEW FROM MY DESK . . .

The premise of this chapter is that disciplined, regularly scheduled work is the key to success; a little work on most days throughout the term is more productive than concentrating all of the effort at crunch time. I have observed that students who do best in their programs tend to adopt the following habits. They

- begin studying in the first week of class;
- manage time and physical demands efficiently, including the unforeseen ones;

- attend all classes, sit near the front, and take notes;
- do all the assigned readings and take notes from them;
- maintain an ongoing list of new vocabulary;
- relate their work to the content and objectives of the course;
- communicate regularly with their instructors, in person or via email;
- gather all available information about assignments and examinations;
- network with fellow students to review lectures and assignments and to share clinical experiences.

STARTING THE RIGHT WAY

College and university programs present students with heavy schedules that include both courses and clinical rotations. Courses often require a large number of readings and assignments. Assignments are generally due in clusters rather than spread equally across a term or semester, adding to the pressure. As a result, it is important when beginning a program of study to ensure you have mechanisms in place to handle the time and physical demands that will be placed on you.

First, ensure that your **physical supports** are in place. Optimally, you should have a dedicated office space, preferably a room of your own. In choosing the space, consider whether you need quiet to work or whether you are one of those who can easily block out distractions. You should ensure you have shelf space for books, plus a filing cabinet for course papers and journal articles. The 'archaeological' system of filing – that is, piles on the desk and floor that are added to as new materials come in – is a terrible time-waster and stressor when something must be found.

Then there are your **social supports**. Make sure you have a discussion with the significant others in your life, especially if you live with them. You will need their understanding when you have to cancel social occasions, as well as their assistance to take up day-to-day responsibilities you won't have time for. The time for these negotiations is before you start your studies, not in the middle when you – and they – are stressed by your workload. It is unwise to test your relationship by assuming they will be understanding and helpful in a situation with which they, too, are unfamiliar.

Finally, take advantage of your **institutional supports**. Does your institution have a writing centre or academic success centre that you are eligible to use? If so, make sure you use it. Professional writers, including your professors when they publish, regularly ask each other to be their readers. Why shouldn't you also benefit from having a trained eye look over what you've written? If that type of institutional support isn't available to you, draw on your fellow students, and reciprocate – our eye for our own work is sharpened by critiquing that of others. Draw also on your significant others as readers, and don't forget to reward their kindness with a kind word or deed of your own. Reading and commenting on an academic paper is not everyone's idea of a fun evening.

As soon as you receive your academic and clinical schedule, give serious consideration to how you will **manage your time**. Remember that the schedule you are given does not include the time you will need for reading, writing, study, travel, or simply the rest of your life. Don't assume, because you may in general be a good time manager, that everything will somehow get done on time. The work you are undertaking is new. It is easy to underestimate the amount of time you will need to keep up with your course readings. This is especially true during your first term in a program.

A strategy that many find helpful is to map out a large calendar sheet for the term and hang it in your work space. Colours are helpful to indicate different types of work: scheduled classes, tutorials, clinical rotations; assignment and test dates; blocks of time dedicated to reading, writing and study. Don't forget to include social occasions and small rewards for your hard work, such as a nice dinner out at mid-term or a weekend away at the end of term. The calendar is intended to reduce your stress, not add to it, so if you find you are not able to follow the schedule you set, be flexible about making changes to reflect the reality you are experiencing.

Choosing times to schedule for study and writing needs some thought. Base your decisions not only on what times are available to you but also on what times are most efficient for you. Are you sharpest in the morning, or are you a night owl? Are you able to read while in transit to classes or clinical?

The next step in starting the right way involves reading your course outlines a number of times and doing it carefully. Concentrate especially on the instructor's description of the course and its objectives, that is, what the instructor wants you to come away with from the course. Highlight the key words and phrases. The time you spend doing this will reap you great benefits in that crucial time at the beginning of a course when you are overwhelmed with new information. It will also bear fruit as the term goes on and the words you highlighted keep popping up in your classes and readings.

This is especially true of any theoretical frameworks instructors mention in the course description. For many students, learning to understand and use theory is the most challenging part of their studies. If this is you, early familiarity will attune you to the multiple dimensions of theoretical concepts. It will assist in developing your overall understanding of the theory and your ability to apply it in your assignments.

AS THE WEEKS GO BY . . .

Some useful study habits

- Take advantage of your biological clock and work on the most difficult subject at your best times.
- Study unlike subjects back to back, with a short activity break between (e.g., a ten-minute walk or a household chore).
- Within a study block, be realistic about how long you can concentrate. Most people are capable of a 45- to 50-minute burst of activity, followed by a 10–15 minute break.
- If your eyes are drooping tiredly shut, go take a 20-minute nap, have a stretch and a drink of water, and come back to work refreshed.
- If possible, test yourself with copies of old tests and exams.
- Join a study group; participate actively in any online discussion boards that are part of your courses.

- If you have a question or don't understand something, communicate with your instructor through email or class discussion boards, or take advantage of their office hours and visit in person, or ask your question at the end of class.

Building study notes

Many students do not concentrate serious attention on taking notes during classes, in the mistaken belief that everything they need to know for tests and exams will be on the instructor's handouts (e.g., PowerPoint slides). Often they also fail to make a connection between the lectures and the expectations of their writing assignments. As a result, these students don't do as well as they could.

Instructors use their lectures to provide important information only partially covered by handouts or bulleted points on a slide. They also use lectures to relate the content of individual lectures to the wider content and objectives of the course (the ones you so carefully highlighted in the course outline and periodically refer back to).

Take lecture notes with a view to ideas, not just facts. The following suggestions will help you to:

- develop your critical thinking skills;
- write better assignments; and
- write better exams.

Record

Know the course outline and take notes on what is important according to the course framework.

- Your aim is to map the main topics and examples discussed, not to transcribe everything.
- Use spacing and visual layout to show the groupings of ideas.
- Be sure to leave wide left and bottom margins on each page for further comments of your own.

You can also look for signals from the lecturer – verbal and non-verbal – to tell you what's important. For example, lecturers show emphasis through their body language and pauses in speaking. Verbal cues include transitions ('I'd like to turn now to...') and breakdowns ('There are three main issues involved here...').

Review (1)

Long-standing research shows that we remember material better if we review it within 24 hours of learning it. Soon after the lecture, while it is still fresh in your mind, reread your notes for sense, accuracy and completeness. If you have made your notes on a computer, now is the time to print them out. Remember to leave wide left and bottom margins on each page. Now pick out key words from your notes and write them in the left margin.

A mistake many students make is to abandon each week's topic as it passes, coming back to their notes only once exam season looms. But a quick review of the entire term's notes and readings once a week – it needn't take long and can be an easy way to ease into a work session – will more than pay for itself at exam time.

Recite

Cover your notes and use the key words in the margins as cues to recite out loud everything you can about the topic, both in the words of the notes and in your own words.

Reflect

Write your reflections about the topic on the lower part of the page. Also write down any questions your notes raise for you. Relate your notes to points in previous lectures or readings and to your upcoming assignment topics. Include your own thinking:

- on the subject;
- on your experiences as a new member of your profession;
- on ways in which you agree or disagree with the ideas of the instructor and the readings.

Review (2)

Before an exam, recite repeatedly, again covering notes and using marginal key words as cues. Think again about how the notes relate to the overall framework of the course. Exam questions will always be framed in such a way as to get you to apply specific facts and ideas to the larger ideas of the course.

Building a personal annotated bibliography

An annotated bibliography is a record of the books and articles you have read on a topic, with a brief comment on the content and usefulness of each. As the number of entries builds, you can subdivide the bibliography by subject. Increasingly, college and university libraries offer free citation software to students, and there are numerous products available commercially. These often feature a bibliography function that allows you to easily maintain an ongoing record of sources you have consulted, along with your brief comment about a source, and what it might be useful for. Whether you build your bibliography using citation software or manually on your own computer, it will be an invaluable resource as your program progresses and the volume of your readings goes up. The act of entering the source serves to improve your memory of it, and the list itself will be invaluable when you are seeking out research materials for future assignments.

Building a vocabulary book

Maintaining an alphabetized vocabulary book not only helps you learn new vocabulary, it is also tremendously helpful for reviewing just before exams or as a source for your assignments. A small notebook or a computer file will do nicely. If a word or term is new, add it to your vocabulary book along with its definition. For clinical terminology, aim for concise, precise definitions. For theoretical terminology, which tends to be complex and multidimensional, leave a large space and make additions to your definition as your lectures and readings add to your understanding. You will find a vocabulary book especially helpful in your first year – as time goes on, you may find yourself needing to make fewer entries.

STUDYING FOR TESTS AND EXAMS

While instructors will change the questions they ask each year on their tests, they will often use a similar structure for the test. Objective questions, short answer, and long answer are the most common testing mechanisms and they require different study strategies.

Objective tests: The most common types of objective test are multiple choice, true/false, and matching exams. They test content knowledge, so when you are studying focus on details and memorize definitions.

- A good strategy is to draw a cluster map with the topic of each week in a balloon and a cluster of points of information around each balloon. Clustered sets of information are easy to remember because they set up mental associations.
- Actively look through your texts and notes for the kind of material that can be answered objectively.
- If possible, get old copies of objective tests to practise on.

Short answer tests: As you review your lecture notes and readings:

- make a list of the most important terms and their definitions; here you will find the vocabulary book you've built throughout the term to be invaluable;
- write down a definition for each term as it was used in the course;
- think of examples to illustrate each term.

Long answer (essay) tests: If possible, review old essay assignments and tests from the course and select a number of questions whose topics seem central to the course. For as many questions as you can, do the following:

- Write a thesis statement that includes the topic and three main points about it.
- Write an outline for each point – the more details of facts, examples, and quotations from readings you can include, the better.
- Write out an essay answer, allowing yourself only as much time as you'll have during the actual exam.

WRITING TESTS AND EXAMS

Before the exam

Cramming through the night before an exam is far from the ideal way to study, not only because it's an inefficient way of learning but also because of the harmful physical effects of too little sleep and too much caffeine consumed to maintain alertness.

- Do your best to get enough sleep the night before.
- Avoid eating fatty or greasy foods the day or night before and have a healthy breakfast that ideally includes fruit, protein and a carbohydrate.
- Make sure you are adequately hydrated.
- Know where the exam is being written and arrive early.
- While waiting to go in, stay away from other students talking about what might be on the exam – it will only increase your nervousness.
- Sit near the front and listen carefully to all instructions given verbally.

Planning your attack

When you get the exam, devote a few minutes to reading it through slowly and carefully.

- Focus on the directions and highlight the key words, including the action verbs that tell you what your answer should do. Are you being asked to compare two things, or to analyze one? Are you being asked to discuss a topic, or define a term? Later in this chapter, you will find definitions of 'Common Essay and Exam Directions'.
- Identify which questions will be easy for you to answer and which will be difficult.
- There are two schools of thought as to which you should answer first. Choose whichever works best for you:
  - o   for many, answering the easy questions first boosts their confidence for tackling the difficult ones;
  - o   others prefer to get the hard ones out of the way first.
- Another approach is to answer the questions that are worth the highest number of marks first. This way, if you run out of time at the end and can't complete everything, you will lose fewer marks. In general, though, do your best *not* to omit questions entirely. A partial answer will always get you more marks than no answer.
- Divide the time available by the worth of each question or section of objective questions. For example, an essay question worth 33% of a three-hour exam should be given one hour. A set of multiple-choice questions worth 10% should get no more than 20 minutes.
- As you complete an answer, check off the question to ensure you don't miss any.
- At the end, reread the whole exam to make sure you've followed all the instructions correctly and haven't left anything out.

- If you finish early, don't leave. At any point, invigilating instructors may be asked questions that they will clarify for everyone, and you may wish to change something as a result. Use the time to improve your answers or to correct errors in spelling, grammar, and punctuation. You can pick up a few extra marks this way.

Answering different types of questions

Objective questions (multiple choice, true/false, matching)

- Read every word of the question carefully – sometimes instructors lay traps for the careless reader.
- Eliminate answers you know to be wrong.
- Eliminate answers that were not included in the subject matter of the course.
- Cover up answers and anticipate the correct answer, then look for it among the choices.
- What to do when you are in doubt:
  - choose the 'best' answer, which is often the answer that uses a word or phrase specific to the course;
  - choose answers with qualifying words (such as some, often, usually, generally, perhaps) in preference to answers with absolute words (such as always, never, only);
  - make an educated guess (unless there is a penalty for wrong answers).
- Check for clerical errors – make sure you marked the answer you intended!

Some myths about multiple choice questions:

- ✗ Instructors most often use 'c' for the correct answer – not true. Instructors don't put the right answer in one position more often than any other.
- ✗ You should never change your answers. Following your first instinct will always lead you to the right answer – not true. All answers should be carefully reviewed and changed if necessary.
- ✗ Always choose the longest answer – not true. Length has no relation to correctness. In fact, instructors sometimes set long, jargon-filled answers to confuse students who don't know the material well.
- ✗ Eating or drinking something in particular (e.g., apple juice) before a test will make you smarter – not true. There are no quick fixes for a failure to maintain an overall healthy diet and lifestyle.

Short answer questions

- Be sure to write enough. Figure on getting one mark for each correct point or detail included in your answer.
- Make sure your answer is related to the general ideas presented in the course.
- Include as many details, facts, or supporting examples as you can.

Long answer (essay) questions

Devote a few minutes to outlining your answer on a blank sheet of paper. Organize your answer by starting with a concise answer to the question. For example, if you are asked 'What are the benefits of breast feeding education?', turn the question into a statement that ends with 'because':

Breast feeding education is beneficial because

1 breast milk is free and readily available;
2 breast-fed infants tend to score higher on a number of developmental tests;
3 there is some evidence that maternal-infant bonding is enhanced with breast-feeding.

Leave enough space between the three points to outline the evidence you will use to support each one.

Long answer questions often ask for comparisons, in order to assess your understanding of two related topics. For example, a question might ask: 'Discuss the differences between disease and illness.' In planning your answer, you would begin with definitions of the two states:

(a) Disease is defined as the biological condition of malfunctioning in the body, medically defined with respect to a genetic, viral, or pathological basis.

(b) Illness is a subjectively defined state of malfunction, broadly associated with physical pain or discomfort or malfunction. It is defined by the individual experiencing it and is not always consistent with the medical diagnosis.

From here you might use the example of an individual with a chronic condition to compare dimensions of the disease diagnosis/treatment with the illness experience.

Say as much as you can, using short paragraphs. Write legibly. Be sure to use the instructor's favourite ideas and phrases.

Take-home exams

Treat these like any other essay assignment. Provide carefully researched and well-constructed answers complete with references.

GLOSSARY OF COMMON ESSAY AND EXAM DIRECTIONS

Clue word	Action required
Analyze	Means to find the main ideas and show how they are related and why they are important; to break material down into its parts, discuss them, and identify how they connect.
Comment on	Means to discuss, criticize, or explain its meaning as completely as possible.
Compare	Means to show both the similarities and differences.
Contrast	Means to compare by showing the differences.
Criticize (critique)	Means to give your judgment or reasoned opinion on something, showing its good and bad points. It is not necessary to attack it.
Define	Means to give the formal meaning by distinguishing it from related terms. This is often a matter of giving a memorized definition.
Describe	Means to write a detailed account or verbal picture in a logical sequence or story form.
Diagram	Means to make a graph, chart or drawing. Be sure you label it and add a brief explanation if it is needed.
Discuss	Means to describe, giving the details, and to explain the pros and cons of it.
Enumerate	Means to list. Name and list the main ideas one by one. Number them.
Evaluate	Means to judge the value of materials for understanding a particular topic; to give your opinion or some expert's opinion of the truth of some expert's opinion or importance of some research results. Tell the strengths and weaknesses, and what it contributes to the topic.
Explain	Means to make clear and understandable to the reader.
Illustrate	Means to explain or make something clear by concrete examples, comparisons, or analogies.
Interpret	Means to give the meaning using examples and personal comments to make something clear.
Justify	Means to give a statement of why you think it is so. Give reasons for your statement or conclusion.
List	Means to produce a numbered list of words, sentences, or comments. Same as enumerate.
Outline	Means to give a general summary. It should contain a series of main ideas supported by secondary ideas and evidence. Omit minor details.

Prove	Means to show by argument or logic that it is true. The word 'prove' has a very special meaning in mathematics and physics.
Relate	Means to show the connections between things, telling how one causes or is like another.
Review	Means to give a survey or summary in which you describe the important parts and critique where needed.
State	Means to describe the main points in precise terms. Be formal. Use brief, clear sentences. Omit details or examples.
Summarize	Means to give a brief, condensed account of the main ideas. Omit details and examples.
Synthesize	Means to combine elements of knowledge into a new structure (e.g., what the relationship is between the traditional hospital model and some new model of acute care).
Trace	Means to follow the progress or history of the subject.

WHEN THE TEST IS RETURNED . . .

For objective and short answer sections, always check the addition of the marks assigned throughout. Markers, who are concentrating hard on the quality of your answers, sometimes slip up on the math.

For essay questions, there isn't always a relationship between the mark and the number of checkmarks an instructor might put as he or she moves down the page. The grade you receive isn't as simply mathematical as with objective testing. Markers are looking for

- reasoning ability;
- factual accuracy;
- relevance of the answer to the question;
- good organization;
- clear, logical writing;
- complete answers.

You may understand why you got the mark you did, or you may not. In that case, take a few days and read the marker's comments carefully once a day, try to match the comments to your answers carefully, and see if you now understand. Writing centres at many institutions will allow you to bring the paper in for help in understanding the comments and ways to improve in future (though they will *not* comment on the mark itself). If, after all this, you are still unclear on the relationship between the mark and the paper, it's time to approach the marker for clarification. But do it respectfully and be prepared to accept the explanation if the marker does not agree to change the mark.

The five least productive things you can say to a marker:

- I'm sure this mark is wrong.
- I worked really hard on this.
- I should get an A because I always come to class.
- I showed it to [fill in the blank: my mother who's a teacher, the writing centre] and they said it was really good.
- I told you what I planned to do and you said it was a great idea.

CRITICAL READING AND THE ITERATIVE WRITING PROCESS

3

OVERVIEW

- First questions
  - What have I been asked to write?
  - Who is going to read this?
- The iterative writing process
  - Get ready
  - Analyze the assignment
  - Do the research
  - Active reading and brainstorming
  - Do an outline
  - Write the draft
  - Revise and edit
  - Proofreading

FIRST QUESTIONS

Professional writers make writing seem easy. Think about newspaper columnists or professional bloggers who publish a story every day, month after month, year after year. But any of them will tell you it's not so. Most famously, the American columnist Gene Fowler is widely quoted as saying, 'Writing is easy; all you do is sit staring at a blank sheet of paper until the drops of blood form on your forehead.'

In this chapter, we begin where any professional writer begins, with two questions: *What have I been asked to write?* and *who is going to read this?*

What have I been asked to write?

Broadly speaking, there are two kinds of writing: description and argument.

Within description, there are two main categories: description and narrative. Description paints a picture of something at a particular point in time and space. For example, clinical notes will describe a patient's presenting symptoms and diagnostic tests. Narrative tells a story across time, such as an experience caring for a patient or a midwife's engagement with a family.

'Argument' is a process in which we apply evidence to support an idea. The end goal of argument is to persuade the reader to accept an idea or act in a certain way. There are many methods by which arguments are developed, and you will find a guide to writing an argument in Chapter 5.

A famous American architect once said that 'Form follows function'. His idea was that an architect should base the design of a building on the purpose or function it is being built to accomplish. This is as true of writing as it is of buildings. Each form of writing, or 'genre', has its own conventions and guiding principles around structure and use of language, depending on the purpose of the genre. Ultimately, our professional, academic and research purposes shape our writing practices, which in turn improve our ability to achieve those purposes.

To sum up, the form for any particular document is determined according to our reason for writing it. If our goal is to report on research, we write in a genre called 'research reporting' using a conventional structure known as 'IMRAD' (more on that in Chapter 8). If our goal is to promote healthy behaviours in the community, we use the genre of 'health education' – materials such as brochures, posters, websites and social media (see Chapter 9). If our goal is to become reflective practitioners, we engage in a genre called 'reflective writing' (see Chapter 11).

Your course instructors will set a wide variety of assignments throughout your program, with several purposes in mind:

- to teach you the forms of writing that are most common in their particular field;
- to help you learn, by asking you to express in writing, the central ideas and facts taught by the course; in other words, your papers have an **evaluative function**; the instructor wants to judge 'how well is this person doing on my course?' and will express the answer as a grade;
- to teach you how to read beyond the course materials and to learn how to read these sources critically (more about that later) – that is, they have a **formative function**: by encouraging you to engage with what others have written, you learn to think more deeply about and engage with your professional community.

So you will be asked to undertake many types of writing that may be new to you, including but not limited to the following:

- literature reviews (such as an annotated bibliography, summary and critique, evidence-based report, or comprehensive review);
- clinical writing (such as clinical portfolios, practice guidelines and interventions, case history and pathophysiology);
- communication in practice settings (such as emails, memos and letters, briefing notes, applications and CVs or résumés);
- reflective writing (such as journals, narratives, personal statements);
- research papers (such as about the history, theory, and ethics of nursing);
- community health promotion and advocacy (such as brochures, websites, social media).

All of these genres are covered in later chapters.

Who is going to read this?

By 'audience', we mean the person or people who will be reading what you wrote. Writing is such a solitary endeavour that it is easy to forget there is a reader on the other end. But you are not writing in a vacuum – someone is out there who does not know what you know, and who will think or act on the basis of what you say. You mediate between the information and what your reader needs to know or be persuaded of. This means everything you write must be clear and persuasive to that audience. In other words, any piece of writing needs to be consciously directed toward its intended audience.

Your audience may be one individual or many. In your professional career, you will need to communicate persuasively with a wide variety of audiences, including your patients and the general public, your professional colleagues in your own and other health fields, health care managers and administrators, government and regulatory bodies, community agencies, and many others.

Based on who their audience is, writers make important choices about form, content, organization, and vocabulary. Here are some questions about audience to consider:

- How large is my audience? Is it an individual or a group (e.g., health team or organization) or the general public?
- What is my relation to the reader? (e.g., am I writing a paper to get a grade in a course? Am I explaining to teenagers why they shouldn't smoke cigarettes? Am I applying for a position? Am I asking a funding agency for a grant?)
- Am I speaking to my reader for myself or on behalf of a group or organization?
- Is my reader expecting this piece of writing? (e.g., is this a course instructor who's asked for this and is going to read it fully and carefully? Or is this a busy administrator or politician I've sent an unsolicited proposal to?)

- How important is my message to the reader? (i.e., how hard will I have to work to get and retain their attention?)
- What does my audience need or want to know?
- What does my audience already know? (i.e., how much do I have to explain to them?)
- What is the reader likely to do with what I've written? (i.e., will they use it as the basis for some decision, such as funding? Will they use it as the basis for some action, such as introducing a new intervention? Will it change their behaviours, such as adopting safe sexual practices?)
- What is the audience's level of general literacy (i.e., what level of vocabulary, tone and diction will the reader understand and respond to?)
- What is the reader's level of health literacy? (i.e., how much medical terminology can I use without defining or simplifying the language?)

THE ITERATIVE WRITING PROCESS

Broadly speaking, the writing process involves the following stages:

- defining the audience, purpose, and form;
- research and organizing/outlining;
- drafting;
- revising for accuracy and style;
- preparing the presentation copy.

Writing is an 'iterative' process; in other words, it involves multiple repetitions of the same process. Each repetition is called an 'iteration' and the end-point of one iteration serves as the start of the next. The iterative process repeats until the desired goal is reached. In writing, the individual iterations combine reading, thinking, writing, and revising. The early iterations consist largely of reading and thinking, with some writing; the latter stages involve some supplementary reading but consist primarily of writing and revising. All iterations involve a lot of intense thinking.

When we go through periods of intense thinking and cognitive activity such as higher education requires, our brains respond in physical ways. The brain is plastic, meaning that particular activities done intensely and/or repetitively will cause changes in the network of neurons. The connections (synapses) between neurons change – new connections are made, existing ones are strengthened or weakened (or broken altogether). In other words, links between ideas are made stronger or weaker such that thinking of one thing will be more or less likely to draw along the other connected idea. This is why, after years of study and writing, our ability to think analytically and efficiently is improved. However, it also means that after individual sessions of study and writing, we may feel tired. The brain needs time to accommodate itself to the new architecture it has constructed and to absorb all its new knowledge and ways of thinking.

Step 1: get ready

- Prepare your writing space. Clear away other projects and lay out the research materials you are starting with.
- For long or multi-section assignments, break the whole task down into stages and assign feasible deadlines for completing each stage.
- Decide on a writing schedule. The 'gold standard' of writing advice is to work on an assignment daily over a period of weeks. And it is true that it is more productive to work for an hour each day than to work for seven hours once a week. This is because long gaps between writing sessions interrupt the thinking process and you have to waste time getting back into it. It's what we all aspire to, and you will find variations of this in any guide to writing (including a number I myself have written). The reality, though, is that it's mainly professional writers and editors like the people who produce these guides who actually have the time to write every day and space assignments out over a period of weeks. Here's what one graduate student in the health professions had to say:

the wise advice of taking little nibbles daily seems never to apply for me. I tend to binge-write based on current academic, clinical, family, and work commitments. Then get really sick a few times and it's game-over. To my endless entertainment I have a book that describes how to manage research in the 'one bite at a time' fashion ... but I haven't read it through yet ... didn't find time!

Do try, though, to work out a schedule that allows you, if not to distribute your writing time widely, at least not to get sick from stress and overwork!

Step 2: analyze the assignment

- Carefully analyze the assignment. Underline or highlight key words and phrases.
- Ask yourself how this topic fits into the overall subject of the course. For example, does it require you to go into depth for a part of the material already covered in class? Does it ask you to apply a theory from the course to an example from your practice experience? An essay assignment expects you to use the concepts and ways of thinking that the course is trying to teach.
- How long is the assignment? Take careful note of the required length. Often instructors will not read anything beyond what they've asked for. (There is a reason for this: it's to prepare you for the professional world, where this is the norm.)

- What kind of paper is this? Does it ask you to integrate theory, research and/or practice? Does it ask you to pick an issue and write about it? Are you going to be interviewing anyone? Will you be incorporating your own life experience, either one in the past or from your current practice?
- Take note of any specific guidelines on how much research outside course readings the assignment asks for.
- Decide how you will focus the topic of the paper. For example, from the broad topic of 'diabetes' you could take any of these directions, depending on which is appropriate to the course:
  o epidemiology of diabetes;
  o the influence of social determinants of health on diabetes;
  o disease management;
  o the illness experience of the patient/family;
  o diabetes management in an acute vs. a home setting;
  o biophysical effects of drug therapy vs. quality-of-life effects of drug therapy.

Step 3: do the research

What kind of sources are you being asked to use? There are a number of types of 'literature' and you may be asked to draw on any or all of them. Most often, though, you will be asked to use articles from 'scholarly journals', also called 'peer-reviewed', 'refereed' or 'academic'. Peer-reviewed means the journal has a policy of having experts in the field evaluate an article before accepting it for publication. How do you know if that's the case? Most (but not all) peer-reviewed journals are listed, by title, in databases such as Ulrich's Periodicals Directory Online. If you don't find the journal listed in Ulrich's:

- Look at the editorial page, where you will find guidelines for authors wanting to submit an article – if the journal uses a peer-review process, it will say there.
- Look for information about the author on the first or last page of an article – he or she should be affiliated with a university or research organization. Be aware, though, that scholarly authors often write to inform the wider public about their research or ideas, so authorship doesn't always mean an article is scholarly.
- The length of the article is also a clue – longer articles (more than ten pages) are usually scholarly.
- Are there a lot of references in the article, at least ten? Some have as many as 100. As you become familiar with the names of scholarly journals and authors, are you seeing these names in the reference list?
- In many library catalogue systems, the initial search page includes a checkbox limiting the search to scholarly/peer reviewed

journals. If you check the box, search results will include only citations to scholarly articles.

- For your search, choose a database that is a major source of scholarly articles, such as MEDLINE or CINAHL or even Google Scholar. Google itself is *not* a reliable way to find scholarly articles. Neither is Wikipedia.

Table 3.1 breaks down the main types of literature and how you might be asked to use them.

For further reading

Cornell University Libraries, Olin & Kris Library. *Distinguishing scholarly journals from other periodicals.* Available at http://olinuris.library.cornell.edu/ref/research/skill20.html

Lederer, N. *Evaluation clues for articles found on the web or in library databases.* Colorado State University Libraries. Available at http://lib.colostate.edu/howto/evalclues.html

Lederer, N. *Popular magazines vs. trade magazines vs. scholarly journals.* Colorado State University Libraries. Available at http://lib.colostate.edu/howto/poplr.html

New York Academy of Medicine. *Grey literature page.* Available at: http://www.nyam.org/library/grey.shtml

Staines, G.M., Johnson, K. & Bonacci, M. (2008) 'Scholarly and popular literature: Making the comparison' in *Social Sciences Research: Research, Writing, and Presentation Strategies for Students* (2nd ed.). Lanham, MD: Scarecrow Press., p. 9.

Weintraub, I. (2006) *The role of grey literature in the sciences.* ACCESS: Brooklyn College Library and AIT E-zine, 10. Available at: http://library.brooklyn.cuny.edu.access/greyliter.htm

Finding the sources

Often it is very helpful to start with Wikipedia, just to get general information about your topic and some starting definitions. For example, for a paper on the history of nursing, you can find an overview of Florence Nightingale's life and times. You can also follow the links at the bottom to sources you can check to see if they are primary (e.g., her diaries) or more scholarly, which you can use for your paper.

Now you are ready to start the serious research. Start with the course readings, and use their reference lists and keywords (located below the title and author information in journal articles) to find more sources. Then use the reference list of each new article as a source to find other articles. Literature review articles and systematic reviews are a great source.

Take note of authors whose names keep turning up – they are likely to be the most important authors on the topic. You'll also see the names of major research institutions repeatedly, such as the Centers for Disease Control and Prevention (CDC).

The next step is to search electronic databases. Consult both general databases like Google Scholar and specialized databases such as Medline, PubMed, CINAHL, Ovid, or the Cochrane Library. The most useful professional index is likely to be MEDLINE (most comprehensive of the approximately 20 health-related databases of Medlar – Medical

Table 3.1 Types of literature

	Scholarly	Professional	Grey	Primary	Popular
Type of publication	Scholarly journals, articles, and books that are usually 'peer-reviewed' or 'refereed' (see below)	Trade and industry journals; professional college guidelines on standards of care, competencies, etc.	1. Reports, government documents, statistical reports, newsletters, bulletins, mission and policy statements; health promotion materials, fact sheets 2. The word 'grey' has nothing to do with quality or colour –it is a name originally given by librarians to reflect the challenge of cataloguing these materials	1. In social sciences and humanities, 'primary' refers to original source material that is closest to the person, period, or idea being studied. 'Secondary' refers to writings about the original sources. (NOTE: In sciences, 'primary' is used to mean peer-reviewed original research published in scientific and scholarly journals. 'Secondary' generally refers to review articles.) May or may not be a published item; can be an artifact, document, recording, video, etc. Health promotion posters and pamphlets would also be considered primary sources	1. Magazines, newspapers, general interest websites 2. Wikipedia and other 'wikis'
Published by	1. Academic institutions (e.g., a university) 2. Organizations that perform original research (e.g., WHO, CDC) 3. Commercial publishers (e.g., Sage)	1. Professional or occupational groups and organizations 2. Regulatory bodies (e.g., RNA, CNA, ANA)	1. Government agencies, research centres, universities, public institutions, non-profit organizations, and associations and societies 2. NOT commercial publishers		1. Commercial publishers 2. Online community of contributors

(Continued)

Table 3.1 (Continued)

	Scholarly	Professional	Grey	Primary	Popular
Purpose	1. To disseminate scholarly knowledge and research 2. The major venue of communication for the science community to present results of current research to colleagues and students	To disseminate professional standards, news about the profession, professional trends, or editorial comment on the profession	1. To provide scholars, professionals and lay readers alike with research summaries, facts, statistics, codes and standards, and other data related to the expertise of the publishing organization 2. To disseminate current information to a wide audience		1. To entertain and inform the public or particular segments of the public 2. To make money for the publisher
Audience	Scholars, researchers, students	Professionals and practitioners within the field	Scholars, professionals and the general public	N/A	General public or a targeted demographic, e.g., golfers or pet owners
Subject matter	Narrow and specific topics related to research, theory or practice in the health and social sciences. Normally consist of an abstract, keywords, introduction, methods, results, discussion, acknowledgments and references	Specific topics relevant to the profession	A wide variety of topics	A wide variety of topics	A broad range of general interest topics intended to entertain and inform, to sell products, or promote a viewpoint

	Scholarly	Professional	Grey	Primary	Popular
Articles written by	Expert researchers with a) academic credentials (e.g., PhD) b) professional credentials (e.g., RN, MD) c) institutional affiliation (e.g., a university or research institute)	Experts on the topic with a) professional credentials such as RN b) institutional affiliation (e.g., a health centre, government, or professional body)	Experts within the organization	A person with direct knowledge of a situation, or a document, etc. created by such a person	1. Popular press: staff or free-lance writers. They may be experts on the topic, or have no prior knowledge at all. Articles often unsigned 2. Wikis (Wikipedia): Anyone. May or may not be an expert; entries can be incomplete or inaccurate
How articles are chosen	Usually go through a formal 'peer-review' process where experts in the field evaluate articles before they are accepted for publication	May be peer-reviewed or may be commissioned by the editor	May be peer-reviewed	N/A	1. Editor decides a topic is timely and assigns a writer OR a writer proposes a topic to an editor 2. Anyone can contribute but the best wikis (such as Wikipedia) enforce ethical and editorial guidelines and rank the accuracy and completeness of entries

(Continued)

Table 3.1 (Continued)

	Scholarly	Professional	Grey	Primary	Popular
Ratio of text to graphics	1. Heavily text-oriented. Articles can be long and dense. Graphic material usually confined to tables and figures 2. Journals usually have plain covers and paper	Heavily text-oriented with tables and graphs, but may also include photos, e.g., of professional events	Usually heavily text-oriented	Highly variable, from fully textual to fully graphic	1. Articles usually brief 2. Glossy paper and colour illustrations 3. Heavy use of creative visuals
Kind of language used	Highly technical and specific to the scholarly field; assumes the reader has the relevant technical background to understand, so there is little explanation of terms	Technical language of the field	Ranges from highly specialized to general	Highly variable	Geared to a wide audience; often no specialty or background knowledge is assumed; language can be very simple or may assume a certain level of education
Funded by	Academic or research institutions; government and other agency grants	1. Professional memberships 2. Advertising	Government or organizational funding	N/A	Sales and advertising revenues
Some important characteristics	1. They always cite sources (at least ten) 2. Reference lists cite other scholars 3. Affiliations of authors listed on the first or last page	1. May cite sources, but not usually as many as scholarly sources 2. Often contain advertising relevant to the occupation	1. Often lack the bibliographic control of scholarly sources, so basic information such as author, publication date or publishing body may not be provided 2. Little or no advertising	Often stored in archives, but may be digitized by the collection that holds the archive and available electronically	1. Do not cite original sources 2. Information may be second or third hand 3. Contain as much advertising as they can sell

	Scholarly	Professional	Grey	Primary	Popular
	4. Most don't include advertising, with some exceptions such as *Science* or *Nature* 5. many are listed in Ulrich's *Periodicals Directory*				
Examples	• *JAMA (Journal of the American Medical Association)* • *Journal of Maternal Child Nursing*	• *Nursing and Midwifery Council Code* • *Registered Nurse Journal*	Publications by • WHO or CDC • HMSO in UK • GPO in US • Queen's Printer in Canada • AGPS in Australia	Personal papers of historical persons such as Florence Nightingale	• *Today's Parent* • *Scientific American* • *Psychology Today*
Use for	1. Your main source for course papers 2. Important source for research and theory	Important for codes, guidelines and practice standards	1. Excellent for facts, statistics and other information or data to give a comprehensive view of the topic 2. As a supplement to scholarly journal literature	To give historical context	1. Only use in special circumstances such as a media analysis 2. Wikipedia is a great starting point for an overview of a topic or a definition. Use the reference list at the end of the entry to find some beginning research materials. But Wikipedia is NOT an acceptable source itself, just an entry point for research

Literature Analysis and Retrieval System). The other essential database for nursing students is CINAHL (Cumulative Index to Nursing and Allied Health Literature). Many college and university libraries offer workshops or online tutorials on how to search these.

Searches of electronic databases may produce a large number of results, even after you have narrowed your search with keywords and Boolean operators (such as 'and'/'or'). At this point, scanning the titles and reading abstracts will help you narrow further still until you get the number you need.

Not all sources are found in electronic databases, though. Some of your sources will be primary, such as the mission statements of your practice setting, or newspaper articles raising issues in health care.

Very important tip: Make up a bibliographic entry before reading a source. After reading, go back and add a few words to say what you might use it for. This saves time later when you are under stress to meet your deadline: 1. You will not forget you've read something and go find it again; 2. You will not have to spend time constructing your reference list because you can just copy-and-paste.

Step 4: active reading and brainstorming

There are two types of reading: **content** and **critical**. We read for content when we want to know how to assemble a piece of furniture, or what the statistics were on coronary disease in 1998. Content reading means reading for information. It employs what we call 'closed thinking'.

Critical reading means reading for idea and argument. We read critically when we want to make judgments about *how* a text is argued and what that argument is. It employs what we call 'open thinking'.

There is also a difference between **passive** reading and **active** reading. We read magazines or social media passively, sitting still as we absorb the content of one article or item and move on to the next. But when we read in order to write, the process becomes active. We physically engage with the material by writing on it and making notes about it. We integrate the activities of thinking and writing into the reading process. It is slower, of course, than passive reading but in fact, over the arc of writing the paper, we save time because we've been building written text right from the start.

The active reading process

- If there is an abstract, read it first to gain a good summary understanding of the article.
- Skim through the article, especially the introduction and conclusion, just to see the names of headings and get a sense of the article's structure. You'll also get a sense of which of the sections will be most relevant for your topic.
- Read the article right through once or twice passively, until you feel you have a good understanding of its contents. Never start copying sentences or passages that look useful without reading the article right through at least once. This is because writers will typically make the same point in a

variety of positions in the article, from different perspectives or in relation to different evidence. It's better to wait until you identify these different iterations of the point and can summarize or paraphrase them using words of your own, rather than just passively copying.

- Pick up a pen or highlighter. Go through the article carefully to underline, bracket or highlight key words, concepts, phrases or sentences. Engage with the material by making marginal notations or jotting down ideas/questions/points related to topic. Pay particular attention to the first sentences of sections and paragraphs – it is in these 'topic sentences' that writers state directly what point is about to be made.
- Read for understanding of their ideas and evidence, as well as to spark your own thoughts and questions about the article and your topic.
- A tip on reading research studies: if you have never taken a course on statistics or research design, skip over the 'Analysis' section that describes the statistical tests the researcher(s) performed to validate their results and establish that they are 'significant'. The significant results are then talked about in the Discussion section.

The second stage of active reading is 'brainstorming', which is a form of free associative writing in which you write down any and all thoughts that occur to you about your paper and the sources. Brainstorming can be done anywhere, even on public transit on the way to school or your practice setting. Don't worry about quality – go for quantity. You can't know whether an idea will turn out to be useful or not, so just get it all down. If you typically suffer from writer's block at the sight of a blank computer screen or paper, you'll find brainstorming especially helpful. No longer will you be starting your draft with that paralyzing blank screen or paper in front of you.

Very important tip: Reading articles in this way is time-consuming and therefore can create stress. Unfortunately, you need to spend extra time learning how to read articles when you are in the early stages of a program. Don't despair – you will get faster at it as you build your knowledge base.

Step 5: do an outline

Whether you are a 'linear' or an 'organic' writer (see Step 6 below), never be tempted to skip the outline stage and jump into writing the draft. The outline is the skeleton of your paper – it's not something you can build in retroactively. A linear writer might prefer a detailed outline, while an organic writer might prefer a sketch of the main points. Whatever kind of outline you prefer, take the time to organize your thoughts and write one.

- What does an outline do?
  - o keeps you on topic;
  - o helps you avoid repetition of ideas or evidence;

- o allows you to check the logic of your argument;
- o allows you to see if you've addressed all parts of the assignment;
- o it's an easy way to see if you've handled the topic adequately or need more points;
- o makes writing the draft much easier;
- o allows you to develop and refine your thesis (if there is one);
- o makes it easy to write your abstract or executive summary (if there is one);
- o allows a professor/colleague/friend to comment and advise you on your work-in-progress. Instructors rarely have time to look at drafts, but many will look at an outline.

Q. How many sections should my paper have?
A. It depends

You will always have an introduction and a conclusion, but the number of sections in the body of your paper will vary. Take a look at the assignment instructions: if the instructor lists specific sections she or he wants, that's how many sections you will have. In this case, you are likely to use section headings (see Chapter 6). Use the instructor's wording for the headings.

If it is an assignment that asks you to discuss a topic within any structure you choose, the answer depends on how many main points you have. There is no 'correct' number, but most people seem most comfortable with having three main points – perhaps it has to do with the primordial human desire for stories that have a beginning, a middle, and an end. You are less likely to use section headings for this kind of paper.

Q. How long should each section be?
A. Just as long as it needs to be

There's a common misconception that every section should be the same length. However, some main points take longer to cover than others. Perhaps there's more evidence to include, or it's a more complicated point, or it's the most important one.

Q. Do I always include a thesis statement? What is a thesis anyway?

'Thesis' is a word left over from the days when Classical Greek rhetoric was a standard part of education systems around the English-speaking world. It is just a way of saying that any piece of writing has to have a sentence (or two or three) that tells the reader what your topic is and what you've got to say about it. That is, it introduces a paper by giving a very brief summary of the content and central idea. I might say:

Midwifery is the best health profession in the world.

That is not good enough, but it does the minimum – my topic is midwifery and I say it's a terrific profession. The problem is, it is not a provable statement. 'Best' is a relative term – what's best for a low-risk pregnancy is not what is best for a high-risk pregnancy, which would involve a team of health professionals. A good thesis makes a limited claim and also summarizes the main points that support it. For example:

> Midwifery is the best option for low-risk pregnancies because research has shown it results in lower maternity care costs, reduced mortality and morbidity related to caesarean and other interventions, lower intervention rates, and fewer recovery complications. (Schlenzka, 1999)

For further reading

Schlenzka, P. (1999). Safety of alternative approaches to childbirth (Doctoral dissertation). Department of Social Work and Sociology, Ferrum College. Cited at http://www.americanpregnancy.org/labornbirth/midwives.html

Sample outline 1: linear outline of an undergraduate nursing dissertation: linear structure

Thesis statement:

> This dissertation analyzes the care of a critically ill child integrating two modules: Caring for the Critically Ill Child (FC3D021) and Professional and Management Issues within Child Health (FC3D022). It will demonstrate an understanding of issues that arise during the care of a critically ill child and his family for Meningococcal Septicaemia (MS), along with management issues such as accountability and frameworks for assessment, and will relate theory and its research to practice.

Introduction:

a. Overview of the dissertation chapters

b. Overview of sources:

  –evidence-based research, theory, legislation, policies 1989–present

  –databases used: CINAHL, Cochrane, SIGN, NICE, DoH, NMC, HPA

Chapter 1: Meningococcal Septicaemia

a. Epidemiology

  –definition

  –prevalence

    –0.5–5 cases per 100,000 population per year worldwide (Milonovich, 2007)

    –higher during winter (SIGN, 2008)

    –25% have previous upper respiratory infection (Hart, 2006)

  –incidence

  –morbidity

  –mortality

b. Pathophysiology

-Meningococci invade = endotoxin = binding protein = activation of macrophages

  -increased vascular permeability

  -pathological vasoconstriction and vasodilation

  -intravascular thrombosis

  -myocardial dysfunction (Pathan et al., 2003)

-causes

  -absence of bactericidal antibodies

  -predisposing factors

-clinical signs and symptoms

  -peticheal rash

  -compensated and uncompensated shock

  -leg pain, cold hands and feet

  -altered mental state, irritability, confusion

-long term effects

  -circulatory failure and septic shock (Donovan, 2010)

  -organ damage, loss of limbs and skin necrosis (NICE, 2010)

  -emotional: nightmares, enuresis and temper tantrums

Chapter 2: Nursing care of the critically ill child

a. Assessment

-ABCDE: Airways, Breathing, Circulation, Disability and Exposure

-obtaining consent (NMC, 2008) (DoH, 2009) (WAG, 2010)

b. Stabilization

-aggressive resuscitation and stabilization

-monitoring for deterioration: PEWS

-importance of close monitoring

c. Treatment

-intravenous ceftriaxone (NICE, 2010)

-blood cultures and meningococcal PCR (SIGN, 2008)

-lumbar puncture if not contraindicated

d. Use of guidelines:

   -Paediatric Early Warning Tools (PEWS)

Chapter 3: Family-centred care (FCC)

a. Definition

   -in health/nursing policies (DoH, 2003) (Haines, 2005) (Moorey, 2010)

b. Continuum scale changes

   -five-part practice continuum tool (Coleman, 2003)

c. Advantages of family presence during invasive procedures

   -parental needs and empowerment

   -sense of closure/grieving process (Cottle et al., 2008)

   -study of nurse perspectives (Perry, 2009)

d. Disadvantages

   -health and safety/risk management

   -may prolong or impede procedures

   -stress for nurses

Chapter 4: The nursing role

a. Clinical governance

   -accountability

   -guidelines

   -competencies

b. Benchmarking

   -six generic skills in caring for the critically ill child

   -current lack of benchmarking

Conclusion

   -summary of dissertation

   -recommendations re

      -universal vaccinaton

      -health education

      -adoption of PEWS

      -role of FCC in critical care

      -adoption of benchmarking

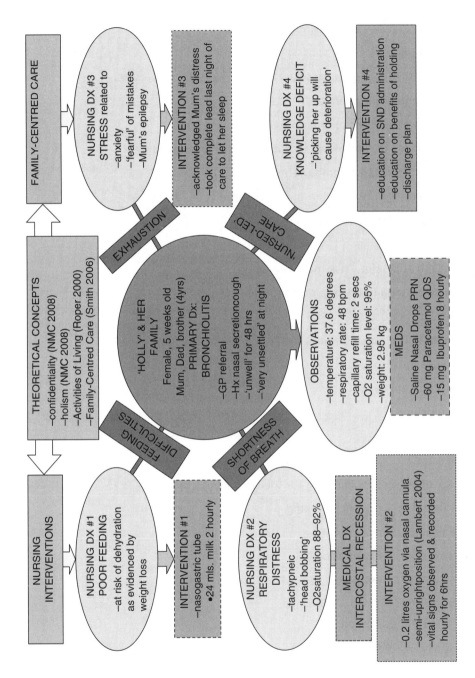

Figure 3.1 Sample outline 2: Concept map of an undergraduate nursing dissertation

Step 6: write the draft

How you write your draft depends on whether you are a 'linear' writer or an 'organic' writer. Linear writers write a document from start to finish. They prefer not to leave a sentence or paragraph until they're comfortable that it's well-written and makes its point. Organic writers will tackle whatever section they have something to say about at that moment. Maybe a course lecture has sparked an idea, or they've found a new article they want to integrate as a source. They build their paper until most of it is written; then they shift to linear writing to make sure everything fits together.

Crafting your paragraphs

If the outline is the skeleton, paragraphs are the muscles that drive the paper forward.

A paragraph is a group of sentences relating to the same idea or topic and forming a distinct part of a piece of writing. There is no 'correct' length for a paragraph. It should be as long as it takes to develop its topic. Generally, however, when a paragraph exceeds a page (double-spaced), you should question whether it covers only one topic or idea, or whether it should be split into more than one paragraph. There are several types of paragraph.

Introductory paragraph: tells the reader the following things. In the dissertation example above, the introductory paragraph functions as a thesis statement. Here, I've broken down its ideas to show how the paragraph introduces the dissertation as a whole:

- the main idea of the paper or section it introduces;
  - o a dissertation on the care of a critically ill child and his family for Meningococcal Septicemia
- the extent or limits of coverage;
  - o based on materials covered in two course modules
- how the topic will be developed;
  - o by discussing issues that arise during the care of the child and his family
  - o by discussing management issues such as accountability and frameworks for assessment
- the writer's approach to the topic;
  - o by relating theory and research to practice.

Body (substantive) paragraph:

- Develops one idea and its supporting evidence.
- Contributes the substance of ideas and information. Most paragraphs are substantive: they develop the argument and deliver the evidence.
- There is no 'correct' length for substantive paragraphs but they are usually three sentences or more but less than a double-spaced page.

Transitional (non-substantive) paragraph:

- Provides a bridge from one section of a paper to another.
- May be as short as only one sentence.
- Ties together what the reader has read so far and what is to come.
- Can be positioned as the concluding paragraph of a section and offer a brief summary of the section.
- Can also be positioned as the introductory paragraph of a new section and offer a preview of its structure and argument.
- Does not contribute any substance to the argument, but functions to move the argument forward.

Concluding paragraph:

- Restates briefly the main ideas of the section or paper.
- Often moves the reader to consider upcoming sections, or may recommend future research or practice.

Types of sentences in paragraphs

Topic sentence:

- Usually the first sentence but may be the second.
- Announces the topic of the paragraph.

Supporting sentences:

- Present facts, reasons, examples, definitions, comparisons, or other evidence to support the central idea of the paragraph.

Concluding sentence:

- Usually the last sentence but may come second-last.
- Sums up the discussion, emphasizes the main point, restates key words of the topic sentence.

Transitional sentence:

- The first (or last) sentence of a paragraph may be a transitional sentence that creates a link to the previous (or next) paragraph.
- Moves the reader from the topic of one paragraph to the topic of the next.

A good paragraph will have **unity** (develops only one idea or point), **coherence** (moves smoothly and logically), and **emphasis** (sentences and words positioned for maximum clarity and impact).

Unity: Means that everything in the paragraph is included to advance one idea or point. Anything that doesn't advance the paragraph's topic should be cut out. The opening sentence (often call the 'topic sentence') tells the reader what the paragraph is about. The middle sentences expand and develop that idea, and the last sentence ties it all up. No extra ideas are introduced and every sentence contributes to the purpose of the paragraph.

Coherence: To be coherent, a paragraph must satisfy several criteria:

a) relevance: every idea relates to the topic;
b) effective order: ideas are arranged in a way that clarifies their logic and/or importance;
c) inclusiveness: nothing vital to the reader's understanding is omitted.

Related to coherence is the stylistic principle of 'flow': the explicit linking words and similarities of grammatical pattern that link sentence to sentence (e.g., repeating key words, using parallel structures). Remember, no matter how clear the connections are to you as a writer, they will not be clear to the reader if they aren't expressed on the page.

Emphasis: This refers to the positioning of important ideas and words for maximum clarity and impact. Emphasis is discussed in detail in Chapter 4.

Step 7: revise and edit

To 'revise' means to 're-vision' – literally, to 're-see' at the **macro level** of overall content, organization, argument, and weight of supporting evidence.

To 'edit' means to sharpen or polish a document. Editing takes place systematically at the **micro level**. At the editing stage, you are attending to the details of language, format, and mechanics:

- **Use of language** refers to word choice, tone, point of view, and logical flow.
- **Format** refers to the physical appearance and arrangement of the document – for example, margin size, font and font size, page numbering, tables and figures, and headings.
- **Mechanics** refers to grammar, punctuation, syntax (sentence structure), spelling, and lack of typographical errors.

A checklist for revision and editing

Structure

- What is the organizing pattern (structure) of your document?
- Does your introduction clearly preview the organizing pattern of your document?
- Does your paper deal with all aspects outlined in the introduction?

- Is your paper broken down into manageable sections which are 'signposted' for your reader (by section headings or topic sentences)?
- Do all parts of your paper flow logically from one to the next with ideas in an appropriate sequence?
- Does the conclusion comprehensively summarize the main points of the paper? Does it offer an evaluation, interpretation, application, or sense of the relevance of your topic? If asked for, does the conclusion include recommendations? Or is it just a generalized statement (such as, 'and therefore midwifery is an important health profession')?

Content

- Reread your draft with your original purpose in mind and ask yourself whether your paper says what you intended it to say and includes all the information that a reader would need.
- Does your document establish common ground with the reader (i.e., explain to the readers why they should care about the problem or issue you've introduced)?
- Does your paper convey a thesis (main argument)?
- Does it identify a significant key issue or issues?
- Does it give a thorough analysis of the key issue's relevant aspects?
- Is your argument convincing because your ideas are fully explained and your arguments are proved by supporting evidence?
- Is there any evidence of unwarranted assumptions or bias that distorts your conclusion?
- Are all your conclusions supported and justified by the evidence?
- Does your argument avoid relying on opinion or generalization?
- Do you substantiate your argument with references to appropriate authorities in the literature?

Style

Check paragraph construction

- Are your paragraphs adequately developed to support your main ideas?
- Are there too many ideas in any paragraph?
- Is there a new paragraph each time there is a shift in topic?
- Are there adequate links/transitions between paragraphs?

Check sentence construction

- Can each sentence be understood on the first reading?
- Are any sentences too short or overly simple?
- Are any sentences too long and complex, with bits awkwardly tacked on or intrusively embedded?
- Is the order of words in any sentence inverted, with the result that the sentence is illogical or difficult to understand?
- Does every sentence coherently follow on from the one before?
- Have you avoided sentence fragments? Run-on sentences? Comma splices? (See the grammar tips in Chapter 4.)

Check the language

- Have you used concrete and specific words rather than abstractions whenever possible?
- Are all your words used correctly and unambiguously?
- Are technical words used appropriately and defined where necessary?
- Have you avoided 'elegant variation' and used terminology consistently so that your reader is never puzzled by varied terminology?
- Have you avoided clichés and language that is too informal?

Mechanics

- Are there any grammar or syntax (sentence structure) errors?
- Are there any punctuation errors?
- Are there any spelling errors? A note on spelling: computerized spell-checkers are a useful tool, but must be supplemented by a careful search of the document. Computerized checkers will not catch homophones (*there, their, they're*) or an incorrect spelling that results in a different but legitimate word (*from, form*).
- Are there any typographical errors?
- Are all reference citations correctly formatted?

When you are in the draft or revision stages, it's always helpful to get feedback from a reader:

- From your professor or marker – take advantage of office hours and extra tutorials.
- From the writing centre at your college or university – take advantage of these highly trained, very sympathetic, expert readers.
- From family and classmates – an objective eye is always helpful. If they don't understand your point, you aren't being clear enough.

Step 8: proofreading

Proofreading the final copy is an important part of the writing process. It requires a lot of concentration and should not be left for, say, 3 am when the assignment is due at 9 am.

To 'proofread' means to ensure that the final, submitted version is completely free of any minor formatting and mechanical errors. It also means ensuring consistency in formatting and mechanics. Especially in long documents (such as a dissertation), it is difficult for the writer to remember that on p. 3 a numbered list was formatted using (1), whereas the numbered list on p. 18 is formatted using 1.

Although some proofreading can be done on your electronic copy of the document, you will need to print out a hard copy to mark up, even if you will be submitting in electronic form.

The challenge in proofreading is maintaining a level of meticulous attention to detail, and keeping the mind focused on individual letters and marks rather than reading to follow the content. Here are some techniques that many writers find helpful:

- Each time you go through the document, read with a single purpose: spelling, punctuation, numbering, heading style, layout of tables and figures, or consistent use of key terms.
- Place a ruler beneath each line as you examine it to keep your eyes from wandering down the page.
- Move up the page from the bottom line to the top.
- Read the document from back to front.
- Read the document aloud to yourself or a colleague who is following a duplicate copy.
- Ask a colleague to proofread for you in exchange for proofreading something of theirs; proofread one final time when you get the paper back.
- Once you find an error or inconsistency in the hard copy, use the find-and-replace function of your electronic file to seek out all other instances of the error.

As someone once said, the only good paper is a done one. Congratulations – you are ready to submit!

BECOMING A
BETTER WRITER 4

This chapter has two objectives:

- to help you develop a personal writing style that is clear, concise and precise;
- to show you how to make choices of structure and language that will help you to respond to any writing task in a style which is appropriate to whatever that task may be.

ELEMENTS OF STYLE

Markers look at four general areas in deciding on a mark for a written assignment:

- how well you have handled the topic and followed the assignment instructions;
- the quality of your ideas and information;
- the way you've organized your paper;
- the quality of your writing style and grammar.

We make a distinction between the **content** and the **style** of a piece of writing. 'Content' refers to *what* is being said; 'style' refers to *how* it is said. Content is the information; everything that is part of the way the information is conveyed makes up the style. A great number of variables, including some intangibles, go together to make up the many styles in which we can write. Once we know what style we want to write in – such as scientific or reflective – writing well means making intelligent choices from amongst the alternatives language makes available to us. These include our choices about sentence structure, grammar, tone, diction, and even punctuation and verbs. To illustrate, these two sentences convey the same content but in very different styles:

- He experienced the ultimate negative surgical outcome.
- He died in surgery.

Sentence structure

Sentence structure (traditionally called 'syntax') refers to the ordering of words and grammatical elements in individual sentences. It is through choices about word order that **emphasis** and **flow**, two important features of a good writing style, are established.

Creating emphasis: When you speak, you have many ways to emphasize words and ideas – body language, gestures, changes in the tone and pitch of your voice – all of which work because your audience can see you (see Chapter 10 on oral presentation). Speech that is completely flat is boring and ultimately hard to understand, and so is writing that gives no sense of relative importance, or 'emphasis'. In writing, the tools for conveying emphasis are syntax and your word choices.

Psychologists have demonstrated that we remember the first and last things we are told significantly better than the material in the middle. Similarly, readers automatically respond to what they read first and last as being most important and most memorable, in other words, the most emphatic. The information that begins a sentence occupies what is called the **topic position**. It both tells the reader what this sentence is about and keeps the reader focused on the perspective, or **point of view**, of the whole paragraph. (Similarly, paragraphs have topic sentences.) Here's an example:

- Poverty is a risk factor for premature morbidity.
- One risk factor for premature morbidity is poverty.

These are both clear, informative sentences about poverty as a social determinant of health, but they establish different points of view. We would expect to see the first sentence in a paragraph about poverty; we'd expect the second in a paragraph discussing risk factors for premature morbidity.

Creating flow: By 'flow', we mean the forward movement of a piece of writing. More specifically, it is the overall coherence and continuity within and among the parts of a piece of writing. Flow is created and maintained by the **repetition** of key words and grammatical constructions, and by the use of **connecting words** that create logical relationships (such as 'and' to indicate addition, or 'therefore' to indicate cause and effect). For example, the beginning of a sentence is an excellent position for linkages between the information of the previous sentence and the information of the new sentence (as I just did here with 'For example,').

Another technique to enhance the forward movement of a sentence is to place the main verb as close as possible to the subject of the sentence. Without the main verb, the reader doesn't know what the subject is doing. A long break in the main thought leaves the reader suspended, neither able to understand the overall meaning of the sentence nor able to fully focus on the information given in the middle. Here's an example:

> **Increased vascular permeability**, where the child can become hypovolaemic due to the reduction in circulating volume, **occurs** where the inflammatory process results in a change in permeability properties of the endothelium.

> **Increased vascular permeability occurs** where the inflammatory process results in a change in permeability properties of the endothelium. The child can become hypovolaemic due to the reduction in circulating volume.

Sentence structures can be simple or complicated:

> *Simple:* The nurse assesses the circulation of the child by examining cardiovascular status.

> *Compound:* The nurse assesses the circulation of the child by examining cardiovascular status, and the nurse also looks for effects of insufficient circulation on other organs.

> *Complex:* Although a child's heart rate can be obtained by a probe, this does not tell the nurse if the pulse is thready, bounding, regular or irregular.

> *Compound-complex:* Although a child's heart rate can be obtained by a probe, this does not tell the nurse if the pulse is thready, bounding, regular or irregular, and thus she or he needs to take a manual pulse rate.

Each structure has its uses, depending on what you are trying to accomplish. Health promotion materials for the general public use sentence structures that are mainly simple or compound. Witness statements, which are legal documents, may use a lot of complex and compound-complex structures. Papers on abstract subjects such as theory, philosophy and ethics may advance complex ideas that require highly complex sentence structures. As a general rule, however, you are more likely to run into trouble with a complicated sentence structure than with a simpler one – when you have a choice, opt for a direct, simple structure.

Another tool for enhancing flow is to organize series of items or ideas using parallel grammatical structures, that is, expressing similar ideas using similar forms. Called **parallelism,** this is one of the most useful organizing techniques in the writer's arsenal. It makes for vigorous, balanced, and rhythmical sentences, and it helps express complex ideas clearly:

- *Eating* huge meals, *snacking* between meals, and *exercising* too little can lead to obesity.

Make sure, though, that the different elements are grammatically the same, unlike in this example:

- *Eating* huge meals, *snacking* between meals, and too little *exercise* can lead to obesity.

Tone and diction

'Tone' refers to the intended emotional impact of a piece of writing. Writing can 'sound' neutral, angry, happy, intimate, concerned, or any other emotion. Notice that these two sentences, which convey the same information, have a very different tone:

My patient had a supportive family which consisted of her husband and two adolescent children.

I was amazed at the bond my patient shared with her loving husband and two teenage kids.

We convey tone through word choice. In writing, 'diction' refers to the specific word choices made by the writer to establish a particular tone. (In speaking, 'diction' has a different meaning: it refers to clarity of speech.) We speak of diction as being formal, informal, or colloquial.

Table 4.1   Levels of diction

Formal	Informal	Colloquial
conducted	did	
examined	looked at	eyed
predicament	problem	a real bind
completed	finished	over with
serendipitous	fortunate	stroke of good luck

Another thing that we need to understand about tone and diction has to do with the history of English. English has two root languages. Prior to the year 1066, Anglo-Saxon was a Germanic language, so different from modern English that it is hardly recognizable as English on first encounter. In 1066, the Normans successfully invaded the island we now call Great Britain and French, a Latin-based language, became the language of the ruling classes. That, combined with the Church's introduction of Latin and Greek as the languages of scholarship and religion, had a profound impact on the English we speak today. It means, among other things, that we often have choices of words to express the same meaning, one derived from Anglo-Saxon and one from Latin or Greek. For reasons that likely have to do with the social history of the two root languages, words of Latin and Greek origin are considered to be more formal and objective in tone. Informal or colloquial diction tends to draw on Anglo-Saxon origins (as do our ripest swear words):

Table 4.2   Latin versus Anglo-Saxon diction

Latin origin	Anglo-Saxon origin
approximately	about
additional	more
cogitate	think
conduct	do
construct	build
demonstrate	show
edifice	building
imbibe	drink
in the absence of	without
in the vicinity of	near
reiterate	say again
necessitate	need
obtain	get
provide	give
solicit	ask for
subterranean	underground
sufficient	enough
utilize	use

Let's consider briefly two kinds of writing about humans that you will be doing and the word choices they entail: writing about the human body and writing about the human experience.

The language of medical sciences, by which we describe the composition and mechanistic functioning of the human body, is not a natural language like English. No baby's first words were ever 'myocardial infarction'. It is a technical language that has been constructed over the past 600 or so years by snipping together bits of Latin and Greek that 'unpack' for the health care professional into very specific information about what has happened [infarct = break] and where [cardio = heart]. It is rigorously precise, unlike the lay term 'heart attack', which inaccurately suggests an external force 'attacking' the heart like a thief in the night:

Table 4.3   A few Latin and Anglo-Saxon health-related terms

Latin origin	Anglo-Saxon origin
ambulatory	can walk
myocardial infarction	heart attack
ischemic event	stroke

It is a mistake to think that writing in formal academic or scientific style means always choosing Latinate diction. Given the complexity of the technical terms of science and medicine, it is usually preferable to seek simpler word choices for other elements in your sentences, both to highlight those important terms and to maintain forward movement. Writing that is overly Latinate is lifeless and challenging for the reader. The example that opened this chapter clearly demonstrates this point:

'He experienced the ultimate negative surgical outcome.'

'He died in surgery.'

There are, however, certain conventions around the use of verbs in research writing that prefer Latinate words – we saw some of them above. For example, in research writing, 'conducted' is preferred to 'did' or 'was done' and 'examined' or 'explored' is preferred to 'looked at'.

Writers are often told to 'avoid medical jargon' in their writing, but what exactly is jargon? For health care professionals, medical language is simply the language they have been trained in, what we call the 'common discourse' of the health sciences professions. It is only when highly technical medical language is used for a wider audience, without explanation or without a need for it, that it becomes jargon.

Unbiased language

Reflective writing and narrative, as we'll see in Chapter 11, are styles that aim to capture multiple dimensions of the human experience. Words that describe the human experience often depend on more than their **denotation** (i.e., their literal meaning). We also depend heavily on their **connotation** (i.e., what they suggest).

Words that seem synonymous are often different in subtle yet important ways. Take these, for example: case, client, patient. All denote a person you are interacting with in your role as a health professional. But a closer look reveals important connotations:

The positive: 'case' is a useful word in medical terminology, because it indicates a focus on those parts of the body that demonstrate signs and symptoms of disease.

The negative: the word is also reductionist, meaning that it reduces complex humans to sets of body parts.

The positive: 'patient' refers to the entire individual, suggesting care that includes all the bio/psycho/social dimensions of health.

The negative: 'patient' suggests waiting, lying passively under the control of experts.

The positive: 'client' empowers the patient into an individual, presumed to have choice and a role in decision-making about their care.

The negative: the person is seen as a consumer, with commercial connotations that are at odds with the sense of compassion that lies at the heart of the healing professions.

Subject, participant. Again, on the surface the words seem synonymous. Both denote an individual who has given informed consent to be scientifically studied. But a 'subject' is one who is ruled by another; a 'participant' is someone working in a partnership role.

Many course instructors, especially in North America, will ask you to use 'APA Style' for your references and formatting, by which they mean the *Publication Manual of the American Psychological Association,* now in its sixth edition (see Chapter 6). In addition to setting uniform standards for scientific communication, the manual also seeks to provide ways, in the words of the editors, to describe individuals with 'accuracy and respect'. By reducing bias in language, your word choices will not suggest any bias against individuals based on sociocultural assumptions about their gender, sexual orientation, ethnicity, disability, or age. Your word choices should:

1 avoid embedded assumptions;
2 be specific;
3 be respectful;

Avoid embedded assumptions: for example, assumptions that certain professions are practised by one gender only. Saying 'lady doctor' suggests that a 'real' doctor is always male; saying 'male nurse' suggests that men cannot be proper nurses. Here are some other common examples:

manpower   vs. staff, human resources
mankind   vs. humanity
mothering   vs. parenting

Pronouns can also perpetuate stereotypes:

✗ Any nurse performing this procedure should protect her hands.

✓ Any nurse performing this procedure should protect his or her hands.

✓✓ Nurses performing this procedure should protect their hands.

Be specific in referring to individuals or groups:

seniors, elderly	older adult
teenager	female adolescent/male adolescent
disabled person	person with a disability
bipolar	person with bipolar disorder
diabetic	person with diabetes
AIDS victim	person living with AIDS
deaf	hearing impaired or profoundly deaf
blind	partially sighted or blind

Well-intentioned euphemisms for persons with disabilities – such as 'special' or 'challenged' – are in fact condescending and shouldn't be used.

In identifying racial and ethnic groups, avoid broad labels such as Asian or Oriental. 'Asian' is wildly inaccurate, as hundreds of distinct racial and ethnic groups inhabit the continent of Asia. Identify the one(s) you are referring to as specifically as you can, such as Chinese-American or Indo-Canadian. 'Oriental' is a word inextricably linked with the history of European colonialism and should not be used except in that context.

Finally, carefully consider whether it is even necessary to include words which emphasize difference. Only include identifiers of disability, sexual orientation, age, or racial/ethnic identity if they are relevant.

Exercise: finding the 'right' word

This is an excellent exercise for reflective papers (see Chapter 11 for a sample) when you are asked to describe and reflect on an experience with a patient or birthing family:

1 Come up with the ten words that best describe the most difficult individual or family you've encountered in your practice setting.
2 Now choose the ten words that best describe the most interesting individual or family you've encountered in your practice setting.

WAYS TO DEVELOP YOUR WRITING STYLE

Be clear

We say that a text is clear if a competent reader who knows the meanings of any technical terms used will understand it on the first reading in the way the writer intended.

Writing can be **unclear**. Unclear passages are challenging and frustrating for readers as they try to figure out what you mean. Here's an example:

> Explanations concerning why cardiovascular training may be beneficial in alleviation of some of the manifestations of FM syndrome include activation of the endogenous opiate system which may function in the modulation of pain (Davis, 2007), physical exercise has been shown to improve mental state (Kerr, 2010), and may provide a sense of purpose and control over a person's body, and provide some resistance of trained muscle to microtrauma (Tremblay, 2008).

There are two clarity problems in this long sentence.

- Word choices that are unclear. 'Explanation' is not a very precise word, ranging in meaning from a verbal explanation to the answers to research questions provided by scientific studies. In this case, 'studies' is what is meant.
- The structure of the sentence. The reader must work through four different grammatical structures. This clarity problem can

occur when we need to include a great deal of information in a sentence. Here, it's a list of the benefits of exercise for improving pain management, mental state, and physical conditioning. For maximum clarity in complex sentences, an effective strategy is to use 'parallel construction', that is, use identical structures to introduce each item in the list. In this case, the little phrase 'on the' will do the job:

✓ A number of studies have examined the benefits of cardiovascular training in alleviating some manifestations of FM syndrome, specifically, **on the function of** the endogenous opiate system in the modulation of pain (McCain, 1996), **on the role of** physical exercise in improving mental state (Kerr, 2010), **and on the resistance of** trained muscle to microtrauma (Tremblay, 2008).

- Writing can be unclear if it is **overly formal.** Trying for 'academic English' can lead to sentences that are dense and difficult to read, but not very informative. They are full of unnecessary words and awkward passive verb constructions. The wish may be to achieve a formal, elegant writing style, but the result is a lifeless writing style that seems to take forever to make its point:

✗ While this may somewhat suggest the ineffectiveness of a passive approach to pain management, it does in no way promote the effectiveness of an active approach. This needs to be achieved through a review of the research literature.

✓ A review of the research literature suggests the effectiveness of an active approach to pain management.

- Writing can be **ambiguous**. Ambigous writing offers at least two different valid interpretations:

The biologists discussed redoing the experiment *for three days.*

Which way did you take the meaning of this sentence? That perhaps the biologists sat in a coffee shop for three days to discuss redoing the experiment? Or that they'd originally done a two-day experiment and were considering making it longer? Or both? The problem here has to do with what we call 'positioning'. In other words, you should place words or ideas that are related to each other as physically close to each other as possible. By placing the 'three days' beside either the authors or the experiment, we link it to whichever one we want:

✓ *For three days the biologists* discussed redoing the experiment.

✓ The biologists discussed *taking three days to redo the experiment.*

Exercise: interpret the meaning created by each variation in positioning

Only one patient took the medication at dinner.

One patient *only* took the medication at dinner.

One patient took *only* the medication at dinner.

One patient took the medication *only* at dinner.

Be concise

Conciseness is a high information-to-words ratio in a text. The opposite of conciseness is wordiness. A concise sentence is not necessarily a short one. Conciseness means using exactly the appropriate number of words, whether that is five or 50. But let's start with a short sentence that demonstrates the point perfectly:

It is certain that needs will increase.

Here we have seven words. If we highlight the words that express a meaning, we have:

It is **certain** that **needs will increase.** ('will' is included because it is part of the verb)

'It is' and 'that' don't convey any meaning, so why include them? Depending on whether we'd like to emphasize the certainty or the needs, we can rewrite in these ways:

✓ Certainly, needs will increase.

✓ Needs will certainly increase.

If you remove three meaningless words out of every sentence in a ten-page paper, you will have fewer than eight pages, and it will be a much clearer paper.

The opposite of conciseness is wordiness, where we use words that repeat what other words already say, or where we simply use more words than are necessary:

✗ A large number of athletes practise some type of a warm-up activity prior to exercising. The goal of warming-up is to prepare the athlete physiologically and psychologically for exercise.

✓ Many athletes warm up to prepare physically and mentally for exercise.

Table 4.4   Wordiness versus conciseness

Original	Revision
a large number of athletes	many athletes
practise some type of a warm-up activity prior to exercising	warm up
the goal of warming-up is to prepare the athlete	to prepare
physiologically and psychologically	physically and mentally

Here is a list of common wordy phrases along with shorter ways to express the same meaning:

a number of	several
appears to be	seems
at the present time	now
at the same time as	while
at this/that point in time	now/then
conducted a study that looked at	studied
due to the fact that	because
for the reason that	because
if conditions are such that	if
in a timely manner	promptly
it is often the case that	often
of a large size	large
on condition that	if
prior to the present time	ago
utilize, utilization	use
was variable	varied
were responsible for	caused

For example:

> ✗ A definition that can be employed usefully, according to LaPlante et al. (1993), states that 'assistive technology...'

> ✓ LaPlante et al. (1993) state that 'assistive technology...'

Next, reduce redundancy:

blue in colour	blue
but rather	but *or* rather
consensus of opinion	consensus
general consensus	consensus
during the process of	during
first and foremost	first
in conjunction with	with
just a few	a few
necessary condition	condition
not unless	unless
one and only	only
only if	if
very few, very rarely	few, rarely

Finally, omit altogether wordy phrases or sentences that fulfil no useful purpose, such as these:

- It is evident that this term is associated with much ambiguity. Many concepts and ideas come to mind upon first hearing this phrase; however, a true grasp of its meaning is quite difficult to establish.

- In this connection the statement can be made that ...
- It is a fact that ...
- It is emphasized that ...
- It is interesting to note that ...

✗ The modern techniques of molecular biology now allow those interested in exercise biochemistry to investigate the regulation and expression of genes that are altered by exercise.

✓ The modern techniques of molecular biology allow biochemists to investigate the regulation and expression of genes altered by exercise.

✗ *It has been established that* slow oxidative fibres *which are rich in mitochondria* can utilize lactate as a fuel.

✓ *Mitochondria-rich* slow oxidative fibres can utilize lactate as a fuel.

Be precise

Precision refers to being exact rather than vague, and specific rather than general:

✗ The profits of No-Name Pharmaceuticals *rose dramatically last year.*

✓ The profits of No-Name Pharmaceuticals *increased 13% in fiscal 2011.*

✗ This paper examines pain management techniques for our rapidly aging population.

✓ This paper examines pain management techniques in elder-care institutions in three urban UK settings.

Avoid ambiguous words (i.e., words with multiple meanings in the context). For example, *as, since,* and *while* are words with both deductive and temporal meanings. They may be making a link of causal relationship, or of relationship in time. If using one of these words will leave the reader in doubt as to which meaning you intend, use a more precise word:

Word:	Causal relationship	Temporal relationship
as	because	at the same time as, when, during
since	because	ever since, after
while	even though, although	at the same time as, when, during

Vague:

We replaced the surgical dressing *as* the incision had healed.

Precise:

We removed the surgical dressing *because* the incision had healed.

We removed the surgical dressing *when* the incision had healed.

Vague:

Since she modified her sodium intake, her blood pressure improved.

Precise:

Because she modified her sodium intake, her blood pressure improved.

After she modified her sodium intake, her blood pressure improved.

Vague:

While we made a case for increased funding, our agency's funding was cut.

Precise:

Although we made a case for increased funding, our agency's budget was cut.

At the same time as we were making a case for increased funding, our agency's budget was cut.

Avoid unnecessary qualifiers:

- ✗ This paper *attempts to explore* the relationship between harm reduction initiatives and rates of homelessness in Vancouver.

Why be hesitant? You are exploring, not just trying to.

- ✓ This paper *explores* the relationship between harm reduction initiatives and rates of homelessness in Vancouver.

Use specific numbers and percentages:

- ✗ Almost half of the participants were drawn from a single setting.

- ✓ Forty-eight percent of the participants were drawn from a single setting.

- ✗ In this study, coaches sometimes reported that their athletes use visual imagery to prepare for competition.

- ✓ In this study, 20% of coaches reported that their athletes use visual imagery to prepare for competition.

Be careful that potentially vague words like 'significant', 'important', 'meaningful', 'unique' are used precisely. 'Unique', for example, means 'the only one of its kind'. It does not have degrees:

- ✗ Smith's study uses the most unique approach our public health nurses had ever seen.
- ✓ Smith's study uses an approach previously unknown to our public health nurses.

If something is 'important' or 'interesting', we must know to whom it's important or interesting, and specifically why:

- ✓ Smith's (2005) findings on carious lesions in childhood (<5 yrs.) will be important for public health nurses working in agencies that serve low income clients.

Avoid vague words such as 'good' that have no precise meaning.

Avoid intensifiers like 'very', 'really', 'actually'. They add nothing to the meaning of the sentence:

- ✗ Tracheal intubation is *actually* the best method of securing the upper airway.
- ✓ Tracheal intubation is the best method of securing the upper airway.

Avoid useless words like 'exist'. If it didn't exist, you couldn't write about it.

- ✗ There *exists* a large body of literature to support this suctioning technique.
- ✓ A large body of literature supports this suctioning technique.

THE VIEW FROM MY DESK: GRAMMAR TIPS AND TRAPS

Here are 16 areas of grammar and usage where students most frequently make errors or ask advice about:

1. Avoid errors in agreement

a. Subjects and verbs should agree in number:

- ✗ Recent *discoveries* about the pathophysiological process *reveals* that several cycles are involved.
- ✓ Recent *discoveries* about the pathophysiological process *reveal* that several cycles are involved.

✗ The *effect* of the social funding cuts *were* clear to all.

✓ The *effect* of the social funding cuts *was* clear to all.

b. Nouns and pronouns should agree in number:

✗ A *nurse* is free to express *their* opinion.

✓ A *nurse* is free to express *his or her* opinion.

✓ *Nurses* are free to express *their* opinions.

c. Pronouns should agree with each other:

✗ Once *one* has decided to take the course, *you* must keep certain policies in mind.

✓ Once *you* have decided to take the course, *you* must keep certain policies in mind.

A note on the pronoun 'one': This pronoun is rarely used now in North American English, where its use seems awkward and old-fashioned. Students sometimes overuse 'one', in the belief that it is a sign of good academic writing style:

✗ If *one wants* to pass the course, *one has* to write the exam.

✓ If *you* want to pass the course, *you* have to write the exam.

✓ *Students who* want to pass the course *have* to write the exam.

2. Watch for irregular plurals

A number of words in common use within the health sciences are nouns of foreign origin (usually Latin or Greek) that do not have standard English endings for singular and plural. Make sure you get them right:

- -on endings: criterion, phenomenon

criterion (sing.) vs. criteria (pl.); phenomenon (sing.) vs. phenomena (pl.):

✓ One new language *criterion was established* for internationally educated nurses.

✓ Six new language *criteria were established* for internationally educated nurses.

- -um endings

datum (sing.) vs. data (pl.).

(✓) Not even one piece of *datum was found* to support this conclusion. [*correct but rare*]

✗ The *data was insufficient* for the authors to draw a conclusion.

✓ The *data were insufficient* for the authors to draw a conclusion.

medium (sing.) vs. media (pl.):

✓ The gel *medium is* prepared for the electrophoresis machine.

✓ The *media have* a large impact on body image among pre-teen girls.

- -x endings

appendix (sing.) vs. appendices (pl.)
index (sing.) vs. indices (pl.)

3. Don't use sentence fragments

A 'sentence fragment' is a group of words that is punctuated to look like a sentence (i.e., it begins with a capital letter and ends with a period), but doesn't fulfil the requirements of a complete sentence. A complete sentence must contain both a subject and a predicate (verb). The subject is what (or whom) the sentence is about, while the verb tells something about the subject or expresses an action. In this next example, there is no subject. We do not know who needs to know about the regulations:

✗ All of these regulations should be made aware.

✓ Midwives should be made aware of all these regulations.

Also, a complete sentence must contain at least one 'independent clause', that is, a group of words that stands by itself as a complete thought. In this example, the second part doesn't make sense on its own:

✗ We poured the acid into a glass beaker. Being the only material impervious to these liquids.

✓ We poured the acid into a glass beaker, which is the only material impervious to these liquids.

✓ Because it is the only material impervious to these liquids, we poured the acid into a glass beaker.

Note: Many people have been told that it is wrong to begin a sentence with 'because'. However, it is perfectly correct when it is introducing a subordinate clause.

4. Deconstruct run-on sentences

A sentence should express only one central idea. In a run-on sentence, one idea 'runs on' into a second. In this next example, the first idea is expansion of home care and the second is what made it possible:

✗ Home care has been expanding tremendously over the past decade partly due to technological advances that enable treatments to be a part of the home setting which at one time could only be performed within the hospital environment.

The ideas should each get a sentence:

> ✓ Home care has expanded tremendously over the past decade. This increase is partly due to technological advances that now make more treatments possible in the home rather than the hospital environment.

It is a common misconception that any long sentence is a run-on sentence. Some sentences need to be long because the single idea they express is complicated or the sentence includes a list.

5. Don't use vague pronouns

Make sure that pronouns such as 'it' and 'this' refer to something specific. 'It is' and 'There are' beginnings not only add meaningless words to a sentence, they can also create confusion. In this next example, what does 'it' refer to? The ischaemic heart disease or the hypertension? It could mean either one:

> ✗ Hypertension is an established risk factor for the development of ischaemic heart disease. *It* is also present in many patients who develop stroke.

> ✓ Hypertension is an established risk factor for the development of ischaemic heart disease. *Hypertension* is also present in many patients who develop stroke.

> ✗ In the report *they* suggest that moderate exercise is better than no exercise at all.

> ✓ The *authors* of the report suggest that moderate exercise is better than no exercise at all.

6. Avoid dangling modifiers

Make sure that a modifying phrase or clause doesn't 'dangle' without the subject it is intended to modify. Here, the first example implies that the pain was doing the manipulating. The second implies that the hobbies go to school:

> ✗ By manipulating the lower back, *the pain* was greatly eased.

> ✓ By manipulating the lower back, *the physiotherapist* greatly eased the pain.

> ✗ When not going to school, *my hobbies* range from athletics to automobiles.

> ✓ When *I* am not going to school, my hobbies range from athletics to automobiles.

7. Avoid squinting or misplaced modifiers

A modifying phrase or clause is said to 'squint' if it applies equally to two different parts of a sentence. Make sure the modifier clearly refers to the element you want it to. In the following example, is the council advising at regular intervals, or should the physicians be administering the drug at regular intervals?

- ✗ The council advises physicians **at regular intervals** to administer the drug.
- ✓ The council advises physicians to administer the drug **at regular intervals.**
- ✓ **At regular intervals,** the council advises physicians to administer the drug.

A 'misplaced' modifier (usually an adverb) is positioned so that it changes the meaning of the sentence. This classic example raises the image of an older gentleman climbing through a window:

- ✗ I could see my grandfather coming through the window.
- ✓ Through the window, I could see my grandfather coming.

8. Use commas correctly

a. The grammar rule is to use a comma before the final 'and' in a series of three or more:

- ✓ Many studies indicate favourable results in function, decreased pain, and range of motion.

In scientific writing, however, that final comma is omitted:

- ✓ Many studies indicate favourable results in function, decreased pain and range of motion.

It is also frequently omitted when the elements of the series are all short (as in the above example). But if they are long or include an internal 'and', make sure you add the final comma:

- ✓ The Neisseria meningitides bacterium infects the body, causes blood poisoning, changes the functions of certain living organisms, and alters physical and chemical process.

b. Use a comma when you join independent clauses with one of the seven coordinating conjunctions (and, or, nor, but, so, yet, for):

- ✗ Power corrupts and absolute power corrupts absolutely.
- ✓ Power corrupts, and absolute power corrupts absolutely.

Note: In scientific writing, the comma is usually omitted.

9. Avoid common errors in punctuation

a. Do not use a comma to separate subject and verb:

✗ His enthusiasm for the project and his desire to be of help, led him to volunteer.

✓ His enthusiasm for the project and his desire to be of help led him to volunteer.

b. Comma splices

A comma splice is the joining ('splicing') of two independent clauses with only a comma. Here are the rules for avoiding them:

Use a period or semicolon to *separate* two independent clauses, or join them with a subordinating conjunction:

✗ We unpacked our instruments, soon we were ready for the test.

✓ We unpacked our instruments; soon we were ready for the test.

✓ We unpacked our instruments, and soon we were ready for the test.

Use a semicolon as well as a conjunctive adverb to *join* two independent clauses:

✗ Much of the literature advocates stretching preparatory to exercise, however, the mechanisms are not well understood.

✓ Much of the literature advocates stretching preparatory to exercise; however, the mechanisms are not well understood.

These are the most common conjunctive adverbs:

- however
- therefore
- thus
- nevertheless
- accordingly
- as a result
- moreover
- even so
- rather
- indeed
- for example

10. Use semicolons and colons properly

a. Use a semicolon when you join independent clauses without a coordinating conjunction:

✗ Power corrupts, absolute power corrupts absolutely.

✓ Power corrupts; absolute power corrupts absolutely.

b. Use a colon to introduce a list or a long or formal quotation after a complete sentence. Otherwise make the quotation part of the grammar of your sentence:

✗ Taylor (2004) points out that: 'Too many programmes are already underfinanced' (p. 87).

✓ Taylor (2004) points out: 'Too many programmes are already underfinanced' (p. 87).

✓ Taylor (2004) points out that 'Too many programmes are already underfinanced' (p. 87).

11. Capitalize correctly

The names of laws, theories, models, or hypotheses are not capitalized. So you would say 'development theory', 'hegemony', 'patriarchal system'. The only exception is for names that include proper names, such as 'Freudian psychology' or 'Jungian collective unconscious'.

To answer a related question, you would capitalize 'Nursing' or 'Midwifery' if you were referring to the name of a specific department or faculty (e.g., Department of Nursing, School of Midwifery), but not capitalize if you are referring to the field of nursing or midwifery.

12. Avoid incorrect comparisons

'Compared to' is often used incorrectly. It shouldn't be used if the sentence contains a comparative term such as 'higher', 'greater', 'less', or 'lower'. For example:

✗ The serum levels in the control group were **higher compared to** the treatment group.

✓ The serum levels in the control group were **higher than** in the treatment group.

✓ The serum levels in the control group were **high compared to** the treatment group.

Another error is the comparison of items that are unlike each other:

✗ Our **results** are similar to our previous **studies.**

✓ Our **results** are similar to the **results** of our previous studies.

13. Don't use double constructions

This is a form of grammar overkill in which a part of speech is unnecessarily duplicated:

x *Since* the legislation has passed, *therefore* we will have more nurse practitioners.

✓ *Since* the legislation has passed, we will have more nurse practitioners.

✓ The legislation has passed; *therefore,* we will have more nurse practitioners.

x The new procedure was popular with *both* doctors *as well as* nurses.

✓ The new procedure was popular with *both* doctors *and* nurses.

✓ The new procedure was popular with doctors *as well as* nurses.

x The *reason for* the legislation was *due to* the long waiting lists.

✓ The *reason for* the legislation was the long waiting lists.

14. Know the difference between 'that' and 'which'

Both 'that' and 'which' can be used in restrictive clauses, but only 'which' is used in non-restrictive clauses:

Restrictive clauses are used when there at least two similar entities, so the one being referred to needs to needs to be identified.

A thermometer is an instrument.

Here, 'instrument' is so large a category that the sentence is almost meaningless. We need to **restrict** our understanding of instrument to the relevant sub-category by adding a clause:

A thermometer is an instrument **that measures temperature.**

A thermometer is an instrument **which measures temperature.**

Restrictive clauses take either 'that' or 'which' and *do not* use commas.

A non-restrictive clause comes after a noun that has already been defined and identified. The clause does not define the noun; it merely adds information about it. The clause can be omitted without causing confusion:

The thermometer, **which is an instrument for measuring temperature,** is standard equipment for visiting nurses.

Non-restrictive clauses take 'which' and *do* use commas. If the clause comes in the middle of a sentence, there are commas both before and after the clause.

15. Avoid strings of nouns

x This study demonstrated significant bipolar disorder interepisodic phase medication effects.

✓ This study demonstrated significant medication effects in the interepisodic phase of bipolar disorder.

Avoid strings of abstract nouns ending in *-ation, -ness, -ism, -ility:*

✗ This paper will provide an **exploration** of the **rationalization** for the local council's **initiation** of its moms and tots group.

✓ This paper will **explore** the **reasons** why the local council **started** its moms and tots group.

16. Don't be afraid to consult the dictionary

Always check words whose meaning you are not sure of:

✗ Explaining the rationale for treatment can help **distil** patients' fears.

✓ Explaining the rationale for treatment can help **dispel** patients' fears.

✗ During restorative procedures, it is **imperial** for natural functions to be preserved.

✓ During restorative procedures, it is **imperative** for natural functions to be preserved.

✗ This study must be **revolutionized** to include the traits that are relevant to the older adult.

✓ This study must be **redesigned** to include the traits that are relevant to the older adult.

VERBS AND USING THEM STRATEGICALLY

Verbs are the sentence elements that tell the reader what the action of the sentence is. A verb can be an 'action verb' that shows the subject doing something, or a 'linking verb' that shows the subject existing or experiencing. When there is a choice, a verb that expresses action is preferable to one that simply expresses existence:

✗ There **exists** a large body of research on the effects of smoking on morbidity.

✓ A large body of research **has studied** the effects of smoking of morbidity.

Verbs can be simple, or they can be verb phrases, which include a verb and any auxiliaries needed to establish tense (such as 'he **arrived** yesterday' vs. 'he **will arrive** tomorrow'). A special class of verbs is called 'modal verbs', which are a type of auxiliary or 'helping' verb. Auxiliary verbs help complete the form and meaning of main verbs. The principal modal verbs are *can, could, may, might, must, should,* and *would.* They combine with main verbs to express meanings such as ability, possibility, permission, obligation, and necessity:

- Cimetidine ***can improve*** mean fat absorption in adolescents with cystic fibrosis. [ability, present tense]
- At first the phlebotomist ***could not locate*** the vein. [ability, past tense]
- We think we ***may receive*** more funding for our program. [possibility, present tense]
- We thought we ***might receive*** more funding for our program. [possibility, past tense]
- Researchers ***may perform*** tests on human participants only with ethics approval. [permission. Note: to indicate permission, 'can' has become almost interchangeable with 'may', especially in North America.]
- We ***must replicate*** their experiment prior to testing our own method. [necessity]
- We ***should seek*** ethics approval before advertising for participants. [obligation]
- Studying these organisms ***would provide*** insight into their protective mechanisms. [possibility]

Tense

'Tense' is the feature of a verb that locates it in time.

Present tense

We use present tense:

1 To describe something that is happening now:

- Appendix A ***summarizes*** the results of the community needs assessment.

2 To describe published research, articles or books whose conclusions you believe are currently valid and relevant. It doesn't matter whether the publication is recent or centuries old:

- Malone (2003) ***discusses*** nursing care in the context of nested proximities.
- In her *Notes on Nursing* (1860), Florence Nightingale ***includes*** practices for cleanliness and observation of the sick.

3 To indicate a general truth or fact, a general law, or a conclusion supported by research results. In other words, something that is believed to be always true:

- The government ***regulates*** the delivery of health care. [fact]

- For every action there *is* an equal and opposite reaction. [law]
- The study results *demonstrate* that cimetidine *can improve* mean fat absorption in adolescents with cystic fibrosis. [conclusion]

4   To describe an apparatus (because it always works the same way):

- This temperature gauge *gives* an accurate reading in all weather conditions.

5   To state research objectives [note: past tense is also commonly used]:

- The purpose of this study *is* to examine imagery use by birthing mothers.

Simple past tense

We use simple past tense:

1   To describe something that began and ended in the past, e.g., the Methods or Results sections of a research report:

- We *administered* four doses daily to 27 participants for 14 days.
- The transgenic plants *showed* up to eight-fold PAL activity compared to control.

2   To describe previous work on which the current work is based:

- Smith et al.'s (2005) study *collected* data on the drug's effect in a paediatric population similar to ours.

3   To describe a fact, law, or finding that is no longer considered valid and relevant:

- Nineteenth-century physicians *held* that women *got* migraines because they *were* 'the weaker sex,' but current research *shows* that the causes of migraine *are* unrelated to gender.

Note the shift here from past tense (discredited belief) to present (current belief).

4   To state research objectives [note: present tense is also commonly used]:

- The purpose of this study *was* to examine imagery use by birthing mothers.

Perfect tense

This tense is formed with the auxiliary ['helping'] verb **have** plus the main verb:

1   Use a present perfect tense to describe something that began in the past and continues to the present:

- Hassanpour *has studied* the effects of radiation treatment since 1982. [and still does]
- Researchers *have demonstrated* a close link between smoking and morbidity rates.

2 Use a **past perfect tense** to describe an action completed in the past before a specific past time:

- Nightingale *had begun* her reforms of nursing practice prior to the Crimean War.

Future tense

Use future tense in outlines, proposals, and descriptions of future work:

- The proposed study *will examine* the effects of a new dosing regimen. Twenty-seven participants *will receive* four doses daily for 14 days.

Progressive tense

Use a progressive tense for an action or condition that began at some past time and is continuing now. It is formed from the auxiliary verb **be** plus a present participle. A progressive form emphasizes the continuing nature of the action:

- I *am collecting* data from three community centres this month.

In places where conciseness is important (such as an abstract or summary), it is common to use a simple verb form instead:

- With this new method, we *are attempting* to demonstrate ...
- With this new method, we *attempt* to demonstrate ...

Active and passive voice

'Voice' is what shows the relationship between the subject and the verb of a sentence. In 'active' (or 'direct') voice, the subject is performing the action. In 'passive' (or 'indirect') voice, the subject is experiencing the action.

The sentence structure that expresses the active voice is subject – verb – object:

- Southern analysis *indicated* a single site of insertion.

Passive voice reverses the order (object – verb – subject). Passive voice is constructed by using a form of the verb **be** followed by a past participle (**-ed**). The phrase 'by [the subject]' is included or it may be implied:

- A single site of insertion *was indicated by* Southern analysis.
- Southern analysis *was performed* [by us] and a single site of insertion *was indicated* [by the analysis].

We use passive voice:

1 To de-emphasize the subject in favour of what has been done:

   - Red or blue outfits **were** randomly **assigned** to competitors in four sports.

2 To discuss background that exists as part of the body of knowledge of the discipline, independent of the current author:

   - Colour **is thought to influence** human mood, emotions and expressed aggression.

As a general principle, use active voice in preference to passive. It is both more direct and more concise:

   ✗ The survey **was conducted by** Chen in 2006.
   ✓ Chen **conducted** the survey in 2006.
   ✗ It is through this paper that the proposed benefits of active exercise for Chronic Lower Back Pain (CLBP) **will be examined**.
   ✓ This paper **will examine** the proposed benefits of active exercise for Chronic Lower Back Pain (CLBP).

Be careful not to shift voice unnecessarily:

   ✗ I **gave** the patient 10cc orally, and 5 more **were given** [by me] intravenously.
   ✓ I **gave** the patient 10cc orally and 5cc intravenously.

FURTHER READING

American Psychological Association. (2010). *Publication manual of the American Psychological Association* (6th ed.). Washington, DC: Author.

Bell, L. (1995). *Effective writing: A guide for health professionals.* Toronto, ON: Copp Clark.

Bennett, J., & Gorovitz, S. (1997). Improving academic writing. *Teaching Philosophy 20*(2), 105–120.

Dixon, B. (1993, April 21). 'What can make scientific papers extremely heavy going is the daunting and lifeless quality of their prose.' *The Chronicle of Higher Education,* Sect. B:5.

Messenger, W. E., de Bruyn, J., Brown, J., & Montagnes, R. (2012). *The Canadian writer's handbook: Essentials edition.* Toronto: Oxford University Press.

Rodman, L. (1996). *Technical communication* (2nd ed.). Toronto, ON: Harcourt Brace Canada.

Ruvinsky, M. (2006). *Practical Grammar: A Canadian writer's resource.* Toronto: Oxford University Press.

Valiela, I. (2001). *Doing Science: Design, analysis, and communication of scientific research.* Oxford: Oxford University Press.

CRITICAL ARGUMENT

5

WHAT IS AN ARGUMENT?

We talked in Chapter 2 about the differences between description and argument, the two broadest categories of writing. An argument is an instrument of persuasion; it must convince the reader to accept its conclusions.

Edward Huth (1990) defines an argument as 'a logically connected series of reasons, statements, or facts used to support or establish a point of view' (p. 56). In other words, we use **evidence** to support an idea or a **claim,** as it is called in formal logic. The purpose of argument is to persuade the reader to accept the claim as true and/or to undertake some action. Notice that in his definition, Huth speaks of establishing or supporting (and to this I would add opposing) a 'point of view' rather than proving a 'fact'. This is because it is very difficult to establish proof either in science or in human experience. Things that were 'known' in the past, for example, have now been thoroughly refuted. Any glance at a nineteenth-century medical text will demonstrate this: Migraine was 'known' to be a disease of women caused by hysteria. We now know that the causes of migraine are not gender-related and are physiological, not psychological. By its very nature, the scientific process is never finished, as the word 'process' itself warns us. We may never know final answers, but we are always in the process of discovering more and refining our understanding. Every piece of research contributes something, fails to contribute something else, and often raises more questions for research than it answers.

Arguments are frameworks designed to help us approach solutions to difficult problems. We need a way to judge the strengths and weaknesses of our options in a logical fashion, and **critical argument** gives it to us. To be 'critical' does not mean to be negative; it means to analyze and evaluate ideas and evidence. The purpose is to understand and express both the strengths and limitations of research, theory or practice, both in terms of its stated purpose and for your own topic. A critical argument is *not* a set of unsupported opinions. For example, the claim that 'nursing is the best profession in the world' cannot be argued. It reflects the writer's personal definition of 'best', which can't be shown to be true for everyone. On the other hand, a claim such as 'nurses are essential members of the health care team' can be argued – by defining in what ways and to whom nurses are essential, and by providing supporting examples.

We can argue **deductively** (start with a general principle and deduce consequences and applications) or **inductively** (start with facts or situations and infer a general principle). We regularly use both deductive and inductive argument in our writing, moving back and forth as needed. Another way to understand deductive and inductive reasoning is this:

- in deductive argument, we advance an idea and then support it with evidence;
- in inductive argument, we start with the evidence, uncovering its strengths and weaknesses, and interpret it to argue for a 'best' position or answer.

Writing that manipulates data technically (such as a lab report) or mathematically (such as statistical analysis) relies on deductive argument, and can in fact establish proof. Here is a simple example of a logical syllogism which proves that one city is larger than another:

Premise 1: London is larger than Toronto.

Premise 2: Toronto is larger than Melbourne.

Conclusion: Therefore, London is larger than Melbourne.

This is a classic example of a 'sound' argument, because it is soundly constructed with a middle term (Toronto) which is equally distributed in the two premises, plus a logical connector (therefore). As long as the premises are true, then the conclusion is true (or 'valid') and we have reasoning that is both sound and valid.

Outside the realm of mathematical proof and syllogisms, however, most written argument is primarily inductive. In reporting on scientific research, for example, researchers use statistical analysis to deduce the statistical significance of their results. Then, however, they argue inductively to interpret the evidence (i.e., the significance) to argue for a particular answer to their research question or objective.

Similarly, you will likely be asked to write about evidence-based practice in one or more of your courses. For example, you may be asked to assess the need for a particular new intervention in your practice setting, to present the best research evidence for and against adopting the intervention, and then come to a conclusion about recommending or not recommending the change.

FEATURES OF WELL-WRITTEN ARGUMENTS

- They are constructed logically. That is, they are coherent and have a logical flow.
- They have an appropriate balance of ideas and evidence.
- They can be summarized clearly and briefly (e.g., in a title, a thesis statement, or an abstract).

Well-written arguments are constructed logically. That is, they are coherent and have a logical flow. We use language to build and strengthen our arguments through:

- **key words and concepts** repeated and added to in a logical sequence;
- **connectors:** transitional words and phrases that establish relationships such as addition, contrast, comparison, causation.

Key words and concepts: As writers, we are intimately familiar with what we are trying to say, and we may sometimes feel that we are boring our readers if we are too repetitive. But in fact, repetition of key words and concepts is an integral part of establishing coherence in argument. In an effort to introduce variety by seeking synonyms for our key words, we can unwittingly introduce confusion for the reader, caused by the fact that synonyms are only sometimes truly synonymous. Often there are subtle differences in meaning; for example, if you are writing a paper about 'empathy', don't switch sometimes to 'sympathy' – they aren't the same and the reader is distracted from your argument to wonder if you've introduced a new concept.

There are other ways of introducing variety in your writing, including in your use of the second key element of argument structure: logical connectors.

Logical connectors are transitional words and phrases that create logical relationships such as addition, contrast, and causation. Table 5.1 classifies the main logical relationships and gives you a variety of synonymous terms to choose from:

Table 5.1   Connecting words and phrases that show logical relationships

To show addition	To compare	To contrast	To give an example	To emphasize
a second point	also	although	for example	above all
again	by comparison	but	for instance	certainly
and	equally	conversely	in fact	chiefly
also	in the same manner	however	in particular	especially
another	in the same way	in contrast	namely	indeed
as well	likewise	by contrast	particularly	in fact

(Continued)

Table 5.1   (Continued)

To show addition	To compare	To contrast	To give an example	To emphasize
besides	similarly	nevertheless	specifically	in particular
first, second ...	than	nonetheless	such as	more importantly
for one thing ...		on the contrary	that is	most importantly
for another				
further		on the other hand	to illustrate	primarily
furthermore		rather	as an illustration	unquestionably
in addition		still		
moreover		though		
next		unlike		
or/nor		whereas		
too		yet		

To restate a point	To summarize or conclude	To indicate logical relationship	To introduce a qualification or concession
again	in conclusion	as a result	admittedly
in brief	in other words	consequently	after all
in effect	in short	for this reason	all the same
in other words	in summary	if...then	despite
in short	that is	since	even if
in simpler terms	therefore	so	even though
that is	to sum up	therefore	frequently
to put it another way		thus	generally
to repeat			in a sense
			in general
			in spite of
			occasionally
			usually
			while it is true that

USING LANGUAGE TO BUILD AN ARGUMENT

Let's see how this key word/connector strategy can operate in your writing. This next example is a sentence from the introduction to a policy analysis. The sentence identifies the main argument (the 'central claim') of the paper, and lists the three factors that the argument will focus on:

> In the late 1990s, several factors led to a reduction in community nursing services: **cuts in government funding, changes in societal attitudes,** and **the new market economy**.

In the body of the policy analysis, the writer develops the same information into a paragraph that advances an argument. Here, the writer creates a causal chain of argument by repeating the **key words** of the introduction, *logically connected* into a sequence of claims and evidence:

> In the mid-1990s, the government was influenced by the model of the **new market economy** *and* [1] sought a rationale for **cutting its funding** of social programs. *Thus,* [2] it took advantage of a recent hardening of **societal attitudes** to accelerate its cuts to these services. *As a result,* [3] **community nursing services** were cut by 10% in 1998, *as compared with* [4] a 5% cut in 1997.

> 1 addition
> 2 causation
> 3 causation
> 4 comparison

Deductive and inductive movement

We spoke above about deductive argument (moves from general to specific) and inductive argument (moves from specific to general), and noted that either of these can be used as an overall strategy for an entire paper, a section, or a paragraph. In writing, this movement is achieved by a steady progression of key words that themselves move from most to least specific (or vice versa). In this final example, you'll see two versions of a paragraph that advances a deductive argument. In the first, there is no logical progression of **key words** and no use of *logical connectors:*

> [1] During the last few decades the interest in **fine particulates** has increased dramatically. [2] Many studies have shown that there are negative effects of **air pollution** on human health. [3] Knowledge is growing about the composition of **air pollution**, mechanisms of toxicity and susceptible populations. [4] **This study** is one of the attempts to understand how **fine particulates and ozone** might interfere with the **autonomic regulation of heart**.

> [1] Although a first sentence should make a fairly broad statement, the key concepts of this sentence are vague: what does 'dramatically' mean? How long is 'a few decades' – 20 years? 50 years?

> [2] This sentence introduces the broader topic of air pollution and human health, which is good, but it would be better to move from broad to specific (air pollution to fine particulates) rather than from specific to broad.

> [3] There are specific details in this sentence, which is good, but the reader is left unsure whether the current study is on air pollution or fine particulates. This is also the third sentence in a row that makes vague statements about the literature (interest; many studies; knowledge is growing).

[4] In this sentence the writer leaps back to the topic of fine particulates. Meanwhile, both ozone and autonomic regulation of heart appear from nowhere.

Finally, let's revise. We'll set up a sequence of **key words** and *logical connectors* to create a persuasive deductive argument that moves logically from broad to specific:

[1]   Many studies (e.g., 1–6) have shown that **air pollution** has negative effects on human health.   [2] *Further*, knowledge is growing about the composition of air pollution, mechanics of toxicity and susceptible populations. [3] *In particular*, a number of recent studies (7–11) have focused on the effects of **fine particulates and ozone**. [4] *However*, no research has been conducted to link **fine particulates and ozone** with the **autonomic regulation of the heart**, *despite* clinical evidence that such a link might exist. [5] *Thus*, **this study** was designed to explore the mechanisms by which **fine particulates and ozone** might interfere with **autonomic regulation of the heart**.

[1–3] The key concepts in the first three sentences move logically, from a broad idea (air pollution and human health) to more specific aspects about our understanding of air pollution (composition, toxicity and susceptible populations), to the particular topic of the study (fine particulates and ozone).

[4]   This sentence identifies (however) a gap in our understanding. It links fine particulates and ozone with the autonomic regulation of the heart. Notice that a reason for conducting the research has been added (the clinical evidence). The original paragraph didn't offer any reason why we would want to investigate these things.

[5]   This sentence makes the final links that connect the study with fine particulates/ozone and autonomic regulation of the heart.

FURTHER READING

Huth, E. J. (1990) *How to write and publish papers in the medical sciences* (2nd ed.). Baltimore, MD: Williams & Wilkins.

HOW TO USE AND ACKNOWLEDGE SOURCES

6

USING SOURCES IN YOUR WRITING

What is our relationship to the sources we use to write our papers? Are they just words written by experts that we sprinkle in often enough to satisfy our markers? If that's all they are, why do those same experts also cite sources? After all, they have no markers to satisfy!

Good referencing is important because it:

* shows the sources you have used in your work;
* enables other people to find the sources you have used;
* supports facts and claims you have made in your work;
* avoids the accusation of plagiarism.

PLAGIARISM

All colleges and universities have policies on plagiarism. Typically, these policies will say that it is an academic offense to represent as your own any portion of someone else's work, whether published or another student's or on the internet. Also, a claim that you didn't know you were committing plagiarism will not be accepted if you 'ought reasonably to have known'. The academic penalties can range from loss of marks in the course to expulsion from the institution.

There are two types of plagiarism: intentional and unintentional. The distinction is in many ways an ethical one. Intentional plagiarists understand that what they are doing is wrong but don't care. They deliberately commit fraudulent actions. Unintentional plagiarists are trying to do the right thing but haven't yet learned the right way to use and acknowledge sources. From a disciplinary point of view, universities and professional bodies apply much heavier penalties to intentional plagiarists. Nonetheless, the minimum consequence may be a grade of zero on the assignment, and the maximum consequence can be a ruined academic or professional career.

Intentional plagiarists: the cheaters

a) Downloading a paper (or parts of several) from the internet, changing a few words, and submitting it with your name as author

   * *The Catch*: plagiarism search engines such as turnitin.com locate the original text and flag the paper for the marker.

b) Paying someone else to write your paper

   * *The Catch*: markers grow suspicious when a student's writing style is noticeably different from previously submitted work or test/exam answers.

c) Borrowing or buying a paper from someone who took the course in a previous year and submitting it with your name as author, sometimes making minor changes

   * *The Catch*: markers maintain files of papers submitted electronically, or they may ask students to submit two printed copies and then return only one.

d) Plagiarizing from yourself: submitting a paper you originally submitted in another course

   * *The Catch*: markers notice that the topic of the paper or the evidence used is irrelevant to the assigned topic or the material covered in their course.

Unintentional plagiarists: the honest mistake

a) Group writing: sometimes students are asked to work on one stage of an assignment as a group (e.g., preparing and delivering a class presentation) and then to work individually on another stage (e.g., writing a paper reflecting on the process of working with the group). Occasionally, students will continue to work as a group to save time and because they are comfortable working together. Each member of the group ends up submitting a paper that is almost identical to the others.
b) Relying too heavily on the words and ideas of published sources.
c) Not acknowledging sources clearly and adequately.

The solution for the first mistake is simple – just make sure you stop working together at the point you're asked to. The second and third honest mistakes, though, represent skills and knowledge that all students need to work to gain. Our next section tells you how to gain them.

HOW TO ACKNOWLEDGE SOURCES (AND HOW NOT TO)

Following the lead of Dr Margaret Procter of the University of Toronto, I'm going to approach the topic of how to use sources through a set of the most common questions and myths around when and where to give references. The text of her widely used advice file on 'How not to plagiarize' is available at www.writing.utoronto.ca/

Doesn't putting in references show disrespect to my professors? They already know where my material comes from because their knowledge is so vast

Your professors do indeed know the literature comprehensively but they got that way the same way you are getting there – by reading and then writing about what they read, carefully citing their sources. They aren't reading your paper in order to be informed by you but to see whether you have read and understood the sources, and can use them to advance an argument about the topic.

Isn't it true that what my sources say doesn't belong to them either? There's nothing original under the sun

When it comes to ideas, we might argue that humanity has been kicking around the same basic ideas since we first stood on two feet, merely articulating them in new ways for each new generation. There's some truth to that statement, but it is the uniqueness of each new set of thinkers' approaches and means of expressing or applying the ideas that makes them original. For example, the French philosopher Michel Foucault was far from the first person to understand that power is unequally distributed within society, but he was the first to express the idea of an unequal power relationship between physicians and patients, and his ideas have greatly influenced modern nursing theorists and ethicists.

Can't I avoid problems just by listing every source in the reference list?

No. Every source in your reference list must be cited in the body of the paper, and every source cited in the body must also be in the reference list. (Note: a reference list is not the same as a bibliography, which contains sources the writer feels will be useful to the reader, regardless of whether they are cited in the body of the paper.)

When most of a paragraph is taken from one source, isn't it enough to put a reference at the end of the paragraph?

No, that's not enough. It suggests to the reader that only the final sentence is derived from the source. Even more confusing is when students mix two or three sources into the paragraph, and then give all the citations together at the end of the final sentence. But there's a larger issue here: If an entire paragraph is just a repetition of what's in a source, where is your input, your idea, your argument?

Having said that, sometimes you do need to write a paragraph that derives from a single source. For example, you may need to summarize the research or ideas of an important research study or practice standard. Or you may need to describe a particular clinical technique, research method, theory, or health promotion campaign. The solution is to make it clear to the reader at the beginning of the paragraph or section exactly what the source is and what you are taking from it.

If I put the ideas into my own words, do I still have to clog up my pages with all those names, dates and page numbers?

It is certainly advisable to paraphrase the ideas of others in your own words wherever possible, both to save space and to let you connect ideas smoothly, but that doesn't make the ideas yours. Whether you are quoting directly, paraphrasing or summarizing, make sure you acknowledge the source, giving a page number whenever possible. Don't worry about the visual appearance of all those citations. You might feel that too many author-date citations break up the flow of sentences and paragraphs, sometimes (if you are citing several works at once) for more than a line. You might feel that they present a challenge to readers, who have to distract their attention from what you are saying in order to absorb citations. In fact, citations do a service to readers by showing them how your ideas are related to those of the experts, and by immediately identifying all the sources of the evidence that supports your ideas.

But I didn't know anything about the subject until I started this paper. Do I have to acknowledge every point I make?

It's always safer to over-reference than to under-reference. When in doubt, cite.

As you learn more, you will learn to distinguish more precisely between specific knowledge that you do need to cite and 'common knowledge' that you don't. It's reasonable to expect anyone in the health professions to know, for example, that infant mortality rates in developed nations have dropped over the last century, or that nurses and midwives are regulated by professional colleges. You can also expect readers to know the common knowledge of society in general, for example, that US stands for the United States or UK for the United Kingdom. Other facts are stated so widely that it would be impossible for you to find the original source, for example, the idea that evidence-based practice is the model used in modern health care. You may feel that you don't yet know whether something is common knowledge in health care or not – again, when in doubt, cite. But if you are seeing the same idea stated by a number of authors without citations, that suggests it's an idea that no one individual has 'ownership' of.

How can I tell what's my own idea and what has come from somebody else?

The key is careful record-keeping. As soon as you pick up a new reading, write up a proper author-date citation in APA or Harvard style at the head of the page on which you make your notes about it. Second, if you copy down (or copy-and-paste) distinctive phrases or sentences, put them into quotation marks, along with the page number, so you can remember later that these are not your words.

So what exactly do I have to document?

a) Quotations

A quotation reproduces the original exactly and encloses it within double quotation marks (not singles); always include the page number in the citation:

> Taylor (2013) recommends that you 'keep your quotations as brief as you can' (p. 77).

The plural of 'p.' is 'pp.': (Taylor, 2013, pp. 110–111).

If the material you are quoting is longer than 40 words (such as when reporting what a patient, client or study participant has said), set it out in what is called a 'block quotation' (see below).

Note: In scientific writing, quotations are very rarely used. Thus, if you are asked to do a summary and critique of a research study, do not quote anything in your description of the study. Paraphrase instead.

b) Paraphrases

We use paraphrases to provide key details from a specific section of a source. To 'paraphrase' is to put information from a short section (less than a paragraph) of the original into your own words, being careful not to change key words and phrases in such a way that the original meaning is oversimplified or changed. In a paraphrase, only about a fifth of the wording should be identical to the original; most of the wording should be yours. Include a page number in the citation. *Note*: the percentage of original wording will be higher in paraphrases of the information in scientific research studies.

c) Summaries

'Summary' is a technique for giving the reader, in a short space, the key ideas and evidence of a lengthy text – from a few paragraphs to an entire article or book. Use a summary when a) you will want to refer back to particular ideas and evidence throughout your paper and/or b) the argument of the whole piece is important to your own argument. A summary captures all the essential information; it does not simply lift sentences and make minor revisions. Here is a technique for writing a summary:

1   Start by reading the source carefully and highlighting the key words, concepts and phrases. Avoid highlighting full sentences or paragraphs. One of the most common mistakes is to choose too many main points to highlight. Think carefully about how much space you have for this summary and be realistic about how much you can and can't include.

2   Then put the original aside while you draft your summary by forming your own sentences to contain them.

3   Next, go back to the original to check that you haven't misrepresented or misunderstood it, then revise as necessary.

4   Make sure that, right at the beginning of your summary, you tell the reader exactly why you are giving it to them – what role does the summary play in your larger paper? What do you hope they'll get out of it?

5   Do not put a citation at the end of each sentence. Instead, use the first sentence or two to state clearly exactly what you are taking from the original. Use the wording of subsequent sentences to reinforce that you are still summarizing. For example:

In the next section, Bowlby's (1954) theory of attachment is summarized and then applied to my practice setting leading a breastfeeding class.

There is an excellent example of a summary in Chapter 12, where you will find a sample student paper about the theory of uncertainty. The last paragraph on p. 185 summarizes an article on the theory of uncertainty, and the first paragraph on p. 186 tells the reader specifically how the theory will be used throughout the paper.

OVERVIEW OF REFERENCING STYLES

In this chapter, to 'reference' means to give full publication details of the sources that are used throughout a paper in a list at the end. To 'cite' or a 'citation' refers to what you write in the actual body of your paper where you want to indicate that a source has been used.

In the same way that English-speaking societies agree that the spelling of the name for a domestic feline is 'cat' rather than 'kat' or 'zbg', scholarly and scientific journals use style manuals to provide a consistent set of rules for acknowledging sources, displaying tables and figures, reporting data, and formatting manuscripts. The comparison isn't completely accurate, because there is only one way to spell cat, whereas there are a number of widely-used styles. But the principle of standardization is the same: if the reader has an expectation that is met, his or her focus on the message of the writing isn't interrupted.

Your instructors may require you to use a particular style in your papers, or may say you can use any style, so long as you use it consistently. The two most widely used styles in nursing and allied health professions are Harvard style and APA style, which is a type of Harvard style.

'Harvard style' is an umbrella term referring to citation styles based on the very first systematic citation style, which was developed at Harvard University in the late nineteenth century. Harvard is a 'parenthetical referencing' style, meaning that author-date or author-title citations are embedded, within round brackets (parentheses), right into the text of a sentence. Author-title citation is most commonly used in the humanities, and author-date citation is most common in the behavioural and social sciences. In medical and pharmaceutical sciences, a numbered-note system called Vancouver style is widely used for papers and research. But for many of the health professions, including nursing, midwifery, public health, and social work, the most widely used author-date style is the *Publication Manual of the American Psychological Association* (APA), currently in its sixth edition. This is especially true in North America. In the UK and Australia, both APA and Harvard style are commonly requested. For this reason, the citation and reference examples given in this chapter are provided in both styles. Because there is no universal Harvard style, the Harvard examples follow the Anglia Ruskin University style guide, available from http://libweb.anglia.ac.uk/referencing/harvard.htm, which is typical of styles in UK higher education. UK students may also wish to consult the publications of the Royal College of Nursing (www.rcn.org.uk) and follow their style, which uses minimal amounts of punctuation. For Australian students, if your college or university has no required style guide of its own, the standard Harvard style manual for Australia is Snooks and Co. (2002), *Style manual for authors, editors and printers*, 6th ed., Milton, Qld.: John Wiley & Sons Australia.

One further, important note is that computerized reference-management software is available for purchase, or may be supplied for free by your university or college library. The big advantage of these products is that they automate much of what is described in the rest of this chapter. They also allow you to change from one style to another with the stroke of a key. They may also allow you to build an ongoing bibliography of useful sources and to maintain them in your account.

APA STYLE

APA style or *the APA Manual* refers to the *Publication Manual of the American Psychological Association,* 6th edition, published by the American Psychological Association in 2010. The APA Manual offers instructions on how to do referencing in your papers but also offers much more and is well worth owning.

A brief tour of the APA Manual . . .

In addition to two lengthy chapters on citing sources and referencing, the manual offers basic guidance on writing, the nuts and bolts of grammar and style (punctuation, spelling, capitalization, abbreviations, numbers, statistics), describes how to use graphic elements (tables, figures, photos, etc.), and includes sample papers that illustrate the style.

Features of APA style

We 'cite' a source in the body of our paper, and we 'reference' it in the list of references that comes at the end of the paper. Citations give the author[s] and date (and often the page number) of the source, but don't give the title, internet address/url or any publication information. Readers will go to the reference list for all the information they need to find the source for themselves.

The in-text citations let readers see immediately who wrote the source, without having to flip back and forth to the reference list. The style also makes it easy to observe who the most important sources in the paper are, because their names appear multiple times. Finally, it lets the reader see when the source was written. In most cases, the research cited will be recent, within the past five years, or perhaps ten. There are many, many exceptions, though, such as for discussions of theoretical frameworks, the history of research in a field, or original groundbreaking sources (e.g., Florence Nightingale or Sigmund Freud).

The style has some disadvantages. Citations can use up a lot of words, which can be an issue when you've been given a page or word limit. The rules for non-academic references, such as government documents and professional standards, are both complicated and unclear. Finally, the citations are spatially intrusive – they can take up a lot of space in a sentence, especially when multiple sources are cited at once. This is unlike numbered-note systems such as Vancouver or CSE (Council of Science Editors), which can neatly contain multiple citations within a range. For example, compare these two citations:

> Recent studies of quality of life (Abernethy, 2009; Baylor & Lee, 2008; Chan, Rosseau, & Brinks, 2012; Tam, 2010) suggest a beneficial role for red wine in reducing stress.

> Recent studies of kidney function [1–4] suggest a beneficial role for red wine in preventing heart disease.

Every source cited in the body of your paper *must* have an accompanying entry in the reference list. Every entry in your reference list *must* be cited at least once in your essay. Note: occasionally you will be asked to provide a 'bibliography'. A bibliography differs from a reference list in that it also includes works for background or for further reading, whether or not they are cited in your paper.

How much should you cite in your papers? Some types of writing require more or fewer than others, but the APA Manual makes the following general recommendation: "The number of sources you cite in your work will vary by the intent of the [paper]. For most [papers], aim to cite one or two of the most representative sources for each key point" (2010, p. 169). I would add to this that it's better to over-reference than to under-reference:

> When in doubt, add a citation.

IN-TEXT CITATIONS IN APA STYLE

1   Citing journal articles: Very often articles have more than one author. So do you always need to write out all their names? Sometimes there are a lot of them, as many as ten or more! The answer is, you don't:

●   For a journal article by **one author**, always give the author's last name (no initials) plus the date. The author name can be given 'directly' (i.e., integrated into the flow of the sentence) or 'indirectly' (i.e., within parentheses). In indirect citations, put a comma after the date.

Direct: Taylor (2013) cautions against using too many direct quotations in-text.

Indirect: One study of student citations (Taylor, 2013) found that most students don't cite often enough.

Indirect: One study of student citations found that most students don't cite often enough (Taylor, 2013).

Cite a page number by adding a comma plus 'p.' (or 'pp.' for pages) plus the number: (Taylor, 2013, p. 8)
Cite a range of consecutive pages this way: (Taylor, 2013, pp. 8–11).
Cite multiple, non-consecutive pages this way: (Taylor, 2013, pp. 3, 6).

- For a work by **two authors**, always give the last names of both authors. *Note*: use the word 'and' in a direct citation; use '&' if it is indirect:

McGillis Hall and Doran (2007) studied nurses' perceptions of hospital work environments and found several systemic issues.

A recent study of hospital work environments revealed several systemic issues (McGillis Hall & Doran, 2007).

- For a journal article by **three to five authors**, give the last names of all the authors the first time you cite them. Note the comma before the final 'and'. In subsequent citations, give only the first author's last name plus 'et al.' or 'and colleagues':

Rates of adverse events in regional hospitals have risen dramatically over the last decade (Affonso, Bain, Colucci, & Doran, 2010). Specifically, rates of medication errors have nearly doubled (Affonso et al., 2010).

or

Specifically, Affonso and colleagues (2010) found that rates of medication errors have nearly doubled.

- For a work by **six or more authors**, give the first author's name only plus 'et al.'

In the recent study by McGillis Hall et al. (2010) . . .

In the sample reference list, you will see that the full list of authors in this case is McGillis Hall, Pedersen, Hubley, Ptack, Hemingway, Watson, and Keatings.
Note: 'et al.' is an abbreviation for a Latin phrase, *et alia*, which means ***and others***. Don't forget the period, and don't forget to add a comma before the date in parentheses:

One recent study (McGillis Hall et al., 2010) . . . .

- For a work with **no author**, use a shortened version of the title in quotation marks. The reference list entry is alphabetized according to the title, which is given there in full (see below).

In a recent smoking cessation campaign, the US National Cancer Institute targeted teens ('NCI Launches,' 2011).

2   If the citation comes at the end of your sentence, the period goes *after* the closing parenthesis:

(Taylor, 2013).

3   Long (*block*) quotations of 40 words or more: Block quotations should be used infrequently, and only if they are there for a clear purpose, such as reporting what a patient or interviewee has said, or introducing a specific item within a Code or Standard that will figure prominently in the paper as a whole. Indent the whole quotation and give the page number in parentheses at the end of the last quoted sentence. The period goes *before* the closing parenthesis:

In her chapter on using sources, Taylor (2013) recommends the following:

In general, keep your quotations as brief as you can. You may consider, for example, quoting an entire paragraph from a particular author because he or she has expressed the idea so well. But if you carefully analyze the paragraph, highlighting the key words and concepts, you'll most likely find that you really need to quote only particular phrases or sentences. (p. 82)

4   If you are citing the same article more than once in the same paragraph, you can drop the date after the first time, as long as no confusion with other articles results. *Note*: This does not apply to citations in parentheses, which must always include a date.
5   Some special cases:

a)   Changes from the source in a quotation: Some changes require no explanation, such as changing the first letter of a quotation to an uppercase or lowercase letter, or changing the punctuation mark at the end of a sentence. However, if you wish to omit material from the middle of a sentence, use three spaced ellipsis points to indicate the position where material was omitted:

Taylor (2013) notes that 'if you wish to omit material . . . use three spaced ellipsis points.'

Use four points to indicate any omission between two sentences. The first point indicates the period at the end of the first sentence quoted:

Taylor (2013) notes that to mark any omission between two sentences, you should 'use four points to indicate. . . . the period at the end of the first sentence quoted.'

If you need to make a minor change to the quoted material in order to fit the flow of the sentence containing the quotation, enclose the changed material in brackets (not parentheses):

The APA Manual (2010) makes the following general recommendation: 'The number of sources you cite in your work will vary by the intent of the [paper]' (p.169).

b) Authors that are groups or organizations: In the reference, the name of the organization occupies the 'author' position. For long names, especially ones that you will be repeatedly citing, include an abbreviation in the first citation and use that subsequently.

Infant mortality rates dropped sharply in rural areas with the introduction of pre-natal counselling (World Health Organization [WHO], 2005). A later study confirmed the drop in infant mortality rates (WHO, 2010).

c) Authors with the same surname: Include the authors' initials along with their surnames in your text.

J. K. Browne (1989) and M. A. Browne (1992) also found . . .

d) Two or more works by the same author[s] in the same parentheses: Arrange by year within the parentheses, mentioning the author name[s] only once, and separate the years with commas.

(National Midwifery Council, 2008, 2009)

e) For works by the same authors in the same year, distinguish the works with the letters a, b, c, etc. Repeat the year each time, separating the years with commas:

Nelson (2007a, 2007b) writes about knowing and understanding in nursing practice.

The year with the letters attached will also appear in your reference list, listed alphabetically by title. See the entries for Nelson in the sample reference list below.

f) When you need to cite two or more works by different authors at the same time, put them into a single set of parentheses, and separate them with semi-colons. List multiple references in alphabetical order (*not* by date):

Recent studies (Deloraine, 2008; Flaubert et al., 2005; Marnier, 2007) have focused on childhood obesity.

g) Citing a web page that gives no author, no year, and no page numbers:

- Move the title to the first position in the reference and give the title, or a shortened version, in the in-text citation.
- Put 'n.d.' (for 'no date') instead of a year.
- Count the number of paragraphs from the beginning of the document, and provide the paragraph number.

h) Citing a work you found cited within another work. For example, you are reading Lowansky, who quotes or paraphrases Kurtz. In your reference list, include *only* Lowansky. In text, give the names of both authors, as follows:

Kurtz's study (as cited in Lowansky, 2010) indicates that . . .

A recent study (Kurtz, as cited in Lowansky, 2010) shows that . . .

i) Personal communications: letters, memos, email, telephone conversations, interviews, etc. These kinds of communication are not listed in your reference list because your readers can't go and find them. Cite them in-text only, as 'personal communications'. If you wish to identify what form of communication was used, do so in the text of the sentence:

In a telephone interview, A. B. Abraham (personal communication, November 10, 2011) described her agency's previous needle-sharps campaigns.

j) Citing course lectures: the APA Manual is not written for students, so it does not cover this case but the following example is consistent with sources that are similar to lectures. For the reference list format, see below. In-text, treat the lecture like any other source, giving the lecturer's name as author plus the year, plus a lowercase letter if you are citing more than one lecture:

(Taylor, 2011a, 2011b)

COMMON REFERENCE LIST EXAMPLES IN APA STYLE

Electronic sources

A great many of your sources will be found online rather than in print versions. Indicate an online source by including either a Digital Object Identifier (DOI) or an URL. The DOI is a number assigned to publications on digital networks that allows click-through access to the reference. Typically, you can find the DOI on the first page of an electronic journal article, near the copyright notice.

Nelson, S. (2005). Staffing, ratios and skill mix: Is there an Australian story? *Nursing Inquiry, 12*(1), 1. doi:10.1111/j.1440-1800.2005.00256.x

When no DOI is available, give the URL of the journal or website home page, *not* the article itself. Do not put a period at the end of the URL

Nelson, S. (2007). Embodied knowing?: The constitution of expertise as moral practice in nursing. *Texto & Contexto Enfermagem, 16*(1), 136-141. Retrieved from http://www.scielo.br/scielo.php?script=sci_serial&pid=0104-0707

- Citing an entire website: You do not need a reference list entry in this case. It is enough to cite the home page address of the site in-text:

The U.S. National Institutes of Health website (http://www.nih.gov/) is a gateway to health information from 27 medical research agencies.

- Electronic mailing lists and other online communities: give the author's name or screen name, followed by the complete date (year, month day), the title of the post, the type of online form in brackets, and the retrieval information:

Jordygirl. (2010, June 8). Re: ethics of cultural sensitivity training [Web log comment]. Retrieved from http://nursingstudentblog.ca/2010/06/ethics_of_cultural

Saunders, S. (2011, December 22). Smoking cessation poster [NUR0000 electronic mailing list]. Retrieved from www.utoronto.ca/nursing/nur0000/message/238

APA style for journal articles

- One author:

McGillis Hall, L. (2003). Nursing staff mix models and outcomes. *Journal of Advanced Nursing, 44*(2), 217-226.

- Two authors:

Schreiber, R., & Nemetz, E. (1992). Pay equity for Ontario's nurses. *The Canadian Nurse, 88*(9), 17-19.

- Three to seven authors:

Tourangeau, A. E., Doran, D. M., McGillis Hall, L., O'Brien Pallas, L., Pringle, D., Tu, J. V., & Cranley, L. A. (2007). Impact of hospital nursing care on 30-day mortality for acute medical patients. *Journal of Advanced Nursing, 57*(1), 32-44.

- More than seven authors:

Doran, D., Haynes, R. B., Kushniruk, A., Straus, S., Grimshaw, J., McGillis Hall, L., Dubrowski, A., . . . Jedras, D. (2010). Supporting evidence-based practice for nurses through information technologies. *Worldviews on Evidence-Based Nursing, 7*(1), 4-15.

- No author: Do *not* list the author as 'Anonymous' unless the work is actually signed that way. Instead, move the title into the first position in the reference.

NCI launches smoking cessation support for teens. (2011, December 5). *NCI News*. Washington, DC: U.S. Department of Health and Human Services, National Institutes of Health, National Cancer Institute. Retrieved from www.nih.gov/news/health/dec2011/nci-05.htm

- Group author, such as an organization, agency, or research group:

National Institute of Child Health and Human Development Early Child Care Research Network (NICHHDECCR). (2005). A day in third grade: A large-scale study of classroom quality and teacher and student behavior. *Elementary School Journal, 105*(3), 305-323.

- A government document, retrieved online: what distinguishes these references is the inclusion of any identifying number assigned by the organization to the report. Place it immediately after the title and before the period.

U.S. Department of Health and Human Services, National Institutes of Health, National Centre for Complementary and Alternative Medicine. (2011). *Yoga for health: An introduction* (NCCAM Publication No. D412). Retrieved from http://nccam.nih.gov/health/yoga/introduction.htm

- Legal materials:

In-text citations for legal materials are the same as any other, giving enough information to help the reader locate the reference entry easily. The references, however, are complicated and are formatted in unique styles that differ from APA. Luckily, you are likely reading the materials, or about them, in a source that itself shows you the way to reference. As a typical reference format, the APA Manual recommends you provide the following:

- The title or name of the case (usually Name v. Name),
- The citation, usually to a volume and page of a book where the published case can be found.
- The precise jurisdiction of the court, in parentheses, including the date of the decision.

Horace v. Ovid, 258 F. 2d. 2314 (W.D.Wis. 1989).

For precise details on formatting legal references, consult the following:

US: Harvard Law Review Association, *The Bluebook: A Uniform System of Citations* (*Bluebook*; 18th ed., 2005).
Canada: McGill Law Review, *Canadian Guide to Uniform Legal Citation* (Montreal: Carswell, 1998, 4th ed). [the *McGill Guide*].
Australia: Melbourne University Law Review Association, *Australian Guide to Legal Citation* (AGLC; 3rd ed., 2010).
UK: Oxford Standard for Citation of Legal Authorities (OSCOLA).

- Magazine article:

Posner, M. I. (1993, October 29). Seeing the mind. *Science, 262,* 673–674.

- Daily newspaper article, no author:

Health-care sector swallowing bitter bill. (1994, September 29). *The Globe and Mail*, pp. A1–A2.

- Course lecture:

Taylor, D. B. (2011a, October 15). Beginning the writing process [Lecture]. In *WRT300: Writing in Health Sciences.* Toronto, Canada: University of Toronto.

Taylor, D. B. (2011b, November 18). Using sources and avoiding plagiarism [Lecture]. In *WRT300: Writing in Health Sciences.* Toronto, Canada: University of Toronto.

APA style for books

- First edition:

Baines, C., Evans, P., & Neysmith, S. (1991). *Women's caring: Feminist perspectives on social welfare.* Toronto, Ontario, Canada: McClelland & Stewart.

- New or revised edition:

Waltz, C. F., Strickland, O. L., & Lenz, E. R. (1991). *Measurement in nursing research* (2nd ed.). Philadelphia: F. A. Davis.

- Edited book

Baumgart, A., & Larsen, J. (Eds.). (1992). *Canadian nursing faces the future* (2nd ed.). St. Louis, MO: Mosby Year Book.

- Book, corporate author:

Institute of Medicine, Committee on Nursing Home Regulation. (1986). *Improving the quality of care in nursing homes.* Washington, DC: National Academy Press.

- Book, corporate author, author as publisher:

American Nurses Association. (1987). *The care of clients with addictions.* Kansas City, MO: Author.

- Book, no author or editor:

ITP Nelson Canadian Dictionary. (1998). Toronto, Ontario, Canada: ITP Nelson.

- Article or chapter in an edited book:

Estabrooks, C. (2001). Research utilization and qualitative research. In J. M. Morse, J. M. Swanson, & A. J. Kuzel (Eds.), *The nature of qualitative evidence* (pp. 275–298). Thousand Oaks, CA: Sage.

In-text citation: (Estabrooks, 2001)

FORMATTING AN APA STYLE REFERENCE LIST

Here you can see how a reference list is formatted. Notice the following:

- The list is entirely double-spaced;
- Each entry has a 'hanging indent,' meaning that the first line starts at the left margin and subsequent lines are indented one tab stop.
- Entries are strictly alphabetical, first by author, then by initials and, if necessary, by title. 'Nothing' comes before 'something' so 'Nelson, S'. comes before 'Nelson, S., & Doran, D'.
- Title information is given in italics, including the volume number after a journal title.
- For journal titles, capitalize all important words (i.e., don't capitalize 'joining' words of four letters or less). For article and book titles, only the following words are capitalized:
  - first word of the title;
  - first word of a subtitle;
  - proper nouns.
- APA uses a lot of punctuation, with periods after every initial and commas between almost all elements that don't take a period. This includes a comma before the final '&' in a list of authors.

SAMPLE REFERENCE LIST IN APA STYLE

Almost, J., Doran, D. M., McGillis Hall, L., & Spence Laschinger, H. K. (2010). Antecedents and consequences of intra-group conflict among nurses. *Journal of Nursing Management, 18*(8), 981–992.

American Nurses Association. (1987). *The care of clients with addictions.* Kansas City, MO: Author.

Baines, C., Evans, P., & Neysmith, S. (1991). *Women's caring: Feminist perspectives on social welfare.* Toronto, Ontario, Canada: McClelland & Stewart.

Baumgart, A., & Larsen, J. (Eds.). (1992). *Canadian nursing faces the future* (2nd ed.). St. Louis, MO: Mosby Year Book.

Collins, S., Voth, T., DiCenso, A., & Guyatt, G. (2005). Finding the evidence. In A. DiCenso, G. Guyatt, & D. Cilisksa (Eds.), *Evidence-based nursing: A guide to clinical practice* (pp. 20–43). St. Louis, MO: Elsevier Mosby.

A day in third grade: A large-scale study of classroom quality and teacher and student behavior. (2005). *Elementary School Journal, 105*(3), 305–323.

Doran, D., Haynes, R. B., Kushniruk, A., Straus, S., Grimshaw, J., McGillis Hall, L., Dubrowski, A., . . . Jedras, D. (2010). Supporting evidence-based practice for nurses through information technologies. *Worldviews on Evidence-Based Nursing, 7*(1), 4–15.

Estabrooks, C. (2001). Research utilization and qualitative research. In J. M. Morse, J. M. Swanson, & A. J. Kuzel (Eds.), *The nature of qualitative evidence* (pp. 275–298). Thousand Oaks, CA: Sage.

Glaser, B. G. (1978a). Basic social processes. In *Theoretical sensitivity: Advances in the methodology of grounded theory* (pp. 93–115). Mill Valley, CA: Sociology Press.

Glaser, B. G. (1978b). Theoretical coding. In *Theoretical sensitivity: Advances in the methodology of grounded theory* (pp. 55–82). Mill Valley, CA: Sociology Press.

Glaser, B. G. (1978c). Theoretical memos. In *Theoretical sensitivity: Advances in the methodology of grounded theory* (pp. 83–92). Mill Valley, CA: Sociology Press.

Health-care sector swallowing bitter bill. (1994, September 29). *The Globe and Mail,* pp. A1–A2.

Institute of Medicine, Committee on Nursing Home Regulation. (1986). *Improving the quality of care in nursing homes.* Washington, DC: National Academy Press.

ITP Nelson Canadian Dictionary. (1998). Toronto, Ontario, Canada: ITP Nelson.

Mays, N., Pope, C., & Popay, J. (2005). Systematically reviewing qualitative and quantitative evidence to inform management and policy-making in the health field. *Journal of Health Services Research & Policy, 10 (Suppl),* 6–20.

McGillis Hall, L. (2003). Nursing staff mix models and outcomes. *Journal of Advanced Nursing, 44*(2), 217–226.

McGillis Hall, L., & Doran, D. (2007). Nurses' perceptions of hospital work environments. *Journal of Nursing Management, 15*(3), 264–273.

McGillis Hall, L., Pedersen, C., Hubley, P., Ptack, E., Hemingway, A., Watson, C., & Keatings, M. (2010). Interruptions and pediatric patient safety. *Journal of Pediatric Nursing, 25*(3), 167–175.

Munhall, P. J. (2012). A phenomenological method. In P. L. Munhall (Ed.), *Nursing research: A qualitative perspective* (5th edition) (pp. 113–175). Toronto, Canada: Jones and Bartlett.

National Institute of Child Health and Human Development Early Child Care Research Network (NICHHDECCR). (2005). A day in third grade: A large-scale study of classroom quality and teacher and student behavior. *Elementary School Journal, 105*(3), 305–323.

NCI launches smoking cessation support for teens. (2011, December 5). *NCI News.* Washington, DC: U.S. Department of Health and Human Services, National Institutes of Health, National Cancer Institute.

Nelson, S. (2005). Staffing, ratios and skill mix: Is there an Australian story? *Nursing Inquiry, 12*(1), 1. doi:10.1111/j.1440-1800.2005.00256.x

Nelson, S. (2007a). Embodied knowing?: The constitution of expertise as moral practice in nursing. *Texto & Contexto Enfermagem, 16*(1), 136–141. Retrieved from http://www.scielo.br/scielo.php?script=sci_serial&pid=0104-0707

Nelson, S. (2007b). When caring is not enough: Understanding the science of pain. *Canadian Journal of Nursing Research, 39*(2), 9–12.

Neufeld, K. (2009). *Health human resources.* Ottawa, Canada: Canadian Nurses Association.

Nursing and Midwifery Council. (2008). *The Code: Standards of conduct, ethics, and performance for nurses and midwives.* London: NMC. Retrieved from www.nmc-uk.org

Nursing and Midwifery Council. (2009). *Record-keeping: guidance for nurses and midwives.* London: NMC. Retrieved from www.nmc-uk.org

Posner, M. I. (1993, October 29). Seeing the mind. *Science, 262,* 673–674.

Taylor, D. B. (2011a, October 15). Beginning the writing process [Lecture]. In *WRT300: Writing in Health Sciences.* Toronto, Canada: University of Toronto Faculty of Nursing.

Taylor, D. B. (2011b, November 18). Using sources and avoiding plagiarism [Lecture]. In *WRT300: Writing in Health Sciences*. Toronto, Canada: University of Toronto Faculty of Nursing.

Taylor, D. B. (2013). *Writing skills for nursing and midwifery students*. London: Sage.

Tourangeau, A. E., Doran, D. M., McGillis Hall, L., O'Brien Pallas, L., Pringle, D., Tu, J. V., & Cranley, L. A. (2007). Impact of hospital nursing care on 30-day mortality for acute medical patients. *Journal of Advanced Nursing, 57*(1), 32–44.

U.S. Department of Health and Human Services, National Institutes of Health, National Centre for Complementary and Alternative Medicine. (2011). *Yoga for health: An introduction*. Washington, DC: Author. Retrieved from http:// nccam.nih.gov/health/yoga/introduction.htm

Waltz, C. F., Strickland, O. L., & Lenz, E. R. (1991). *Measurement in nursing research* (2nd ed.). Philadelphia: F. A. Davis.

Wolff, A.C., Ratner, P. A., Robinson, S. L., Oliffe, J. L., & McGillis Hall, L. (2010). Beyond generational differences: A literature review of the impact of relational diversity on nurses' attitudes and work. *Journal of Nursing Management, 18*, 948–969. doi:10.1111/j.1365-2834.2010.01136.x

IN-TEXT CITATIONS IN HARVARD STYLE

1   Citing journal articles:

- For a journal article by **one author**, always give the author's last name (no intials) plus the date. The author name can be given 'directly' (i.e., integrated into the flow of the sentence) or 'indirectly' (i.e., be placed parenthetically).

Direct: Taylor (2013) cautions against using too many direct quotations in-text.

Indirect: One study of student citations (Taylor, 2013) found that most students don't cite often enough.

Indirect: One study of student citations found that most students don't cite often enough (Taylor, 2013).

Cite a page number by adding a 'p.' (or 'pp.' for pages) plus the number:

Taylor (2013, p. 8) or (Taylor 2013, p. 8)

Cite a range of consecutive pages this way: (Taylor, 2013, pp. 8–11).

Cite multiple, non-consecutive pages this way: (Taylor, 2013, pp. 3, 6).

- For a work by **two, three, or four authors**, always give the last names of all authors, with 'and' before the final name. Note that there is no comma before the 'and':

DiCenso, Guyatt and Cilisksa (2005) lay out the principles of evidence-based nursing.

- For a work by **five or more** authors, give the first author's name only plus a comma plus 'et al.'

One recent study (McGillis Hall, et al., 2010). . . .

2   If the citation comes at the end of your sentence, the period goes *after* the closing parenthesis.

(Taylor, 2013).

3   Long ('block') quotations of 40 words or more: Block quotations should be used infrequently, and only if they are there for a clear purpose, such as reporting what a patient or interviewee has said, or introducing a specific item within a Code or Standard that will figure prominently in the paper as a whole. Indent the whole quotation and give the page number in parentheses at the end of the last quoted sentence. The period goes *before* the closing parenthesis:

In her chapter on using sources, Taylor (2013) recommends the following:

In general, keep your quotations as brief as you can. You may consider, for example, quoting an entire paragraph from a particular article because the author has expressed the idea so well. But if you truly analyse the paragraph, highlighting the key words and concepts, you'll most likely find that you really need to quote only particular phrases or sentences. (p.135)

4   Some special cases:

a)   Authors that are groups or organizations: in the reference, the name of the organization occupies the 'author' position. For long names, especially ones that you will be repeatedly citing, include an abbreviation in the first citation and use that subsequently.

Infant mortality rates dropped sharply in rural areas with the introduction of pre-natal counselling (World Health Organization [WHO], 2005). A later study confirmed the drop in infant mortality rates (WHO, 2010).

b)   Two or more works by the same author[s] in the same parentheses: arrange by year within the parentheses, mentioning the author name[s] only once. Separate the years with semi-colons.

(National Midwifery Council, 2008; 2009)

    c)   For works by the same authors in the same year, distinguish the works with the letters a, b, c, etc. Give the year only once, and separate the letters with semi-colons:

Nelson (2007a; b) writes about knowing and understanding in nursing practice.

The year with the letters attached will also appear in your reference list, listed in the order in which they appear in the text. See the entries for Nelson in the sample reference list below.

    d)   When you need to cite two or more works by different authors at the same time, put them into a single set of parentheses, and separate them with semi-colons. List them in chronological order, that is, earliest date first:

Recent studies (Flaubert. et al., 2005; Marnier, 2007; Deloraine, 2008) have focused on childhood obesity.

    e)   Citing a code of ethics or other or professional regulatory standards.

Nurses and midwives must ensure they gain consent before beginning any treatment or procedure (NMC Code, 2008, Standard 13).

Section 7 of Controlled drugs: amendments to the Misuse of Drugs Regulations 2001 (Home Office, 2005) states that . . .

    f)   Citing a work you found cited within another work. For example, you are reading Lowansky, who quotes or paraphrases Kurtz. In your reference list, include *only* Lowansky. In text, give the names of both authors, as follows:

Kurtz's study (2007 cited in Lowansky, 2010) indicates that . . .

A recent study (Kurtz, 2007 cited in Lowansky, 2010) shows that. . .

    g)   Personal communications: letters, memos, email, telephone conversations, interviews, etc. Most Harvard styles do not include these kinds of communication in the reference list because your readers can't go and find them. Cite them in-text only, as 'personal communications'. If you wish to identify what form of communication was used, do so in the text of the sentence:

In a telephone interview, A. B. Abraham (personal communication, 10 November 2011) described her agency's previous needle-sharps campaigns.

    h)   Citing course lectures: in-text, give the lecturer's name plus the year. See below for the reference format.

(Taylor, 2011a; b)

COMMON REFERENCE LIST EXAMPLES IN HARVARD STYLE

Electronic sources

- For a magazine or journal article accessed on the internet:

Nelson, S., 2007. Embodied knowing?: the constitution of expertise as moral practice in nursing. *Texto & Contexto Enfermagem*, [online] 16(1), pp. 136-141. Available at: <http://www.scielo.br/scielo.php?script= sci_serial&pid=0104-0707> [Accessed 10 December 2011].

- For journal articles accessed through a password protected database from a library:

Wolff, A.C., Ratner, P. A., Robinson, S. L., Oliffe, J. L. and McGillis Hall, L., 2010. Beyond generational differences: a literature review of the impact of relational diversity on nurses' attitudes and work. *Journal of Nursing Management*, [e-journal] 18, pp. 948-969. Available through: Scholars Portal database [Accessed 18 December 2011].

- Electronic mailing lists and other online communities: Give the author's name or screen name, followed by the year, the title of the individual post, the title of the forum, type of online form in brackets, and the retrieval information:

Saunders, S., 2011. 'Smoking cessation poster', *NUR0000 electronic mailing list*, [online] 22 December 2011, Available at: <http://www.utoronto.ca/ nursing/nur1001/message/238> [Accessed 18 December 2011].

Jordygirl, 2010. Ethics of cultural sensitivity training. *University of Toronto Faculty of Nursing student blog*, [blog] 8 April, Available at: <http:// nursingstudentblog.ca/2010/06/ethics_of_cultural> [Accessed 15 April 2010].

Harvard style for journal articles

- One author:

McGillis Hall, L., 2003. Nursing staff mix models and outcomes. *Journal of Advanced Nursing*, 44(2), pp. 217-226.

- Two, three or four authors: include all the authors' names and initials, in the order they appear in the original.

Almost, J., Doran, D. M., McGillis Hall, L. and Spence Laschinger, H. K., 2010. Antecedents and consequences of intra-group conflict among nurses. *Journal of Nursing Management*, 18(8), pp. 981-992.

- more than four authors: include only the first author's name and initials plus 'et al.' plus a comma:

Tourangeau, A. E. et al., 2007. Impact of hospital nursing care on 30-day mortality for acute medical patients. *Journal of Advanced Nursing* 57(1), pp. 32–44.

- no author or editor: if no author is given, use 'Anonymous' in the author position.

Anonymous, 2011. NCI launches smoking cessation support for teens. *NCI News*, [online newsletter] 5 December 2011. Available at: <http://www.cancer.gov/newscenter/pressreleases/2011/SmokeFreeTeenTXT> [Accessed 11 December 2011].

- Group author, such as an organization, agency, or research group:

National Institute of Child Health and Human Development Early Child Care Research Network (NICHHDECCR), 2005. A day in third grade: a large-scale study of classroom quality and teacher and student behavior. *Elementary School Journal,* 105(3), 305–323.

- A government document, retrieved online:

U.S. Department of Health and Human Services, National Institutes of Health, National Centre for Complementary and Alternative Medicine, 2011. *Yoga for health: an introduction,* [pdf] Washington, DC: NCCAM. Available at: <http://nccam.nih.gov/health/yoga/introduction.htm> [Accessed 20 December 2011].

- Legal materials:

For court cases, give the names of the parties (Name v Name), followed by the year in brackets, followed by the Law Reports series (e.g., AC, WLR) with the part number, case number or page reference:

Horace v Ovid [1989] EWCA Crim 689, 1989 WL 104528.

For precise details on formatting legal references, consult the following:

US: Harvard Law Review Association, *The Bluebook: A Uniform System of Citations* (Bluebook; 18th ed., 2005).

Canada: McGill Law Review, *Canadian Guide to Uniform Legal Citation* (Montreal: Carswell, 1998, 4th ed). [the McGill Guide].

Australia: Melbourne University Law Review Association, *Australian Guide to Legal Citation* (AGLC; 3rd ed., 2010).

UK: *Oxford Standard for Citation of Legal Authorities* (OSCOLA).

- Magazine article:

Posner, M. I., 1993. Seeing the mind. *Science,* 262, 673–674.

- Daily newspaper article:

Health-care sector swallowing bitter bill, 1994. *The Globe and Mail,* 29 Sep. pp. A1–A2.

- Course lectures:

Taylor, D. B., 2011a. Beginning the writing process, *WRT300: Writing in Health Sciences.* University of Toronto, unpublished.

Taylor, D. B., 2011b. Using sources and avoiding plagiarism, *WRT300: Writing in Health Sciences.* University of Toronto, unpublished.

Harvard style for books

- First edition:

Baines, C., Evans, P. and Neysmith, S., 1991. *Women's caring: feminist perspectives on social welfare.* Toronto, Ontario, Canada: McClelland & Stewart.

- New or revised edition:

Waltz, C. F., Strickland, O. L. and Lenz, E. R., 1991. *Measurement in nursing research.* 2nd ed. Philadelphia: F. A. Davis.

- Edited book:

Baumgart, A. and Larsen, J. eds., 1992. *Canadian nursing faces the future.* 2nd ed. St. Louis, MO: Mosby Year Book.

- Article or chapter in an edited book:

Estabrooks, C., 2001. Research utilization and qualitative research. In: J. M. Morse, J. M. Swanson and A. J. Kuzel, eds. *The nature of qualitative evidence.* Thousand Oaks, CA: Sage, pp. 44–68.

In-text: (Estabrooks, 2001)

- Book, corporate author, author as publisher:

Nursing and Midwifery Council, 2009. Record-keeping: guidance for nurses and midwives, [online] London: NMC. Available at: <www.nmc-uk. org> [Accessed 5 January 2012].

Personal communications: letters, memos, emails, telephone conversations, interviews, etc.

Most Harvard styles do not include personal communications in the reference list, because the reader cannot retrieve them. Cite them in-text as 'personal communications'. If you wish to identify what form of communication was used, do so in the context of the sentence.

In a telephone interview, A. B. Abraham (2011, pers. com., 10 November) described her agency's previous needle-sharps campaigns.

If you are asked to include personal communications in your reference list, you can use this format:

Abraham, A. B., 2011. *Needle-sharp campaigns.* [telephone] (Personal communication, 10 November 2011).

FORMATTING A HARVARD STYLE REFERENCE LIST

Many of the examples in this section have been compiled into a sample reference list. Here you can see how a reference list is formatted. Notice the following:

- Entries are single-spaced with a double-space between entries.
- Entries are not indented.
- Entries are strictly alphabetical, first by author, then by initials and, if necessary, by title. 'Nothing' comes before 'something' so 'Nelson, S.' comes before 'Nelson, S., & Doran, D.'
- Title information for journals and books is given in italics, but not including the volume number after a journal title.
- For journal titles, capitalize all important words (i.e., don't capitalize 'joining' words of four letters or less). For article and book titles, capitalize only the first word of the title and proper nouns (e.g., Scotland).

SAMPLE REFERENCE LIST IN HARVARD STYLE

Almost, J., Doran, D. M., McGillis Hall, L. and Spence Laschinger, H. K., 2010. Antecedents and consequences of intra-group conflict among nurses. *Journal of Nursing Management,* 18(8), pp. 981–992.

American Nurses Association, 1987. *The care of clients with addictions.* Kansas City, MO: American Nurses Association.

Anonymous, 2011. NCI launches smoking cessation support for teens. *NCI News,* [online newsletter] 5 December 2011. Available at: <http://www.cancer.gov/newscenter/pressreleases/2011/SmokeFreeTeenTXT> [Accessed 11 December 2011].

Baines, C., Evans, P. and Neysmith, S., 1991. *Women's caring: feminist perspectives on social welfare.* Toronto, Ontario, Canada: McClelland & Stewart.

Baumgart, A. and Larsen, J., eds., 1992. *Canadian nursing faces the future.* 2nd ed. St. Louis, MO: Mosby Year Book.

Collins, S., Voth, T., DiCenso, A. and Guyatt, G., 2005. Finding the evidence. In: A. DiCenso, G. Guyatt and D. Cilisksa, eds. *Evidence-based nursing: a guide to clinical practice.* St. Louis, MO: Elsevier Mosby, pp. 20–43.

Doran, D. et al., 2010. Supporting evidence-based practice for nurses through information technologies. *Worldviews on Evidence-Based Nursing,* 7(1), pp. 4–15.

Estabrooks, C., 2001. Research utilization and qualitative research. In: J. M. Morse, J. M. Swanson and A. J. Kuzel, eds. *The nature of qualitative evidence.* Thousand Oaks, CA: Sage, pp. 275–298.

Glaser, B. G., 1978a. Basic social processes. In: *Theoretical sensitivity: advances in the methodology of grounded theory.* Mill Valley, CA: Sociology Press, pp. 93–115.

Glaser, B. G., 1978b. Theoretical coding. In: *Theoretical sensitivity: advances in the methodology of grounded theory.* Mill Valley, CA: Sociology Press, pp. 55–82.

Glaser, B. G., 1978c. Theoretical memos. In: *Theoretical sensitivity: advances in the methodology of grounded theory.* Mill Valley, CA: Sociology Press, pp. 83–92.

Health-care sector swallowing bitter bill, 1994. *The Globe and Mail,* 29 Sep. pp. A1–A2.

Home Office, 2005. Controlled drugs: amendments to the Misuse of Drug Regulations 2001. (Home Office Circular 048/2005) [pdf]. Available at: <http://www.homeoffice.gov.uk/about-us/corporate-publications-strategy/home-office-circulars/circulars-2005/048-2005/> [Accessed 11 December 2011].

Institute of Medicine, Committee on Nursing Home Regulation, 1986. *Improving the quality of care in nursing homes.* Washington, DC: National Academy Press.

ITP Nelson Canadian Dictionary, 1998. Toronto, Ontario, Canada: ITP Nelson.

Jordygirl, 2010. Ethics of cultural sensitivity training. *University of Toronto Faculty of Nursing student blog,* [blog] 8 April, Available at: <http://nursingstudentblog.ca/2010/06/ethics_of_cultural> [Accessed 15 April 2010].

Mays, N., Pope, C. and Popay, J., 2005. Systematically reviewing qualitative and quantitative evidence to inform management and policy-making in the health field. *Journal of Health Services Research & Policy,* 10 (Suppl), pp. 6–20.

McGillis Hall, L., 2003. Nursing staff mix models and outcomes. *Journal of Advanced Nursing,* 44(2), pp. 217–226.

McGillis Hall, L. and Doran, D., 2007. Nurses' perceptions of hospital work environments. *Journal of Nursing Management,* 15(3), pp. 264–273.

McGillis Hall, L. et al., 2010. Interruptions and pediatric patient safety. *Journal of Pediatric Nursing,* 25(3), pp. 167–175.

Munhall, P. J., 2012. A phenomenological method. In: P. L. Munhall, ed. *Nursing research: a qualitative perspective.* 5th ed. Toronto, Canada: Jones and Bartlett, pp. 113–175.

National Institute of Child Health and Human Development Early Child Care Research Network (NICHHDECCR), 2005. A day in third grade: a large-scale study of classroom quality and teacher and student behavior. *Elementary School Journal,* 105(3), pp. 305–323.

Nelson, S., 2005. Staffing, ratios and skill mix: Is there an Australian story? *Nursing Inquiry,* 12(1), p.1.

Nelson, S., 2007a. Embodied knowing?: the constitution of expertise as moral practice in nursing. *Texto & Contexto Enfermagem*, [online] 16(1), pp. 136–141. Available at: <http://www.scielo.br/scielo.php?script=sci_serial&pid=0104-0707> [Accessed 10 December 2011].

Nelson, S., 2007b. When caring is not enough: understanding the science of pain. *Canadian Journal of Nursing Research*, 39(2), pp. 9–12.

Neufeld, K., 2009. *Health human resources.* Ottawa, Canada: Canadian Nurses Association.

Nursing and Midwifery Council, 2008. *The Code: standards of conduct, ethics, and performance for nurses and midwives,* [online] London: NMC. Available at: <www.nmc-uk.org> [Accessed 5 January 2012].

Nursing and Midwifery Council, 2009. Record-keeping: guidance for nurses and midwives, [online] London: NMC. Available at: <www.nmc-uk.org> [Accessed 5 January 2012].

Posner, M. I., 1993. Seeing the mind. *Science,* 262, pp. 673–674.

Saunders, S., 2011. 'Smoking cessation poster', *NUR0000 electronic mailing list,* [online] 22 December 2011, Available at: <http://www.utoronto.ca/nursing/nur1001/message/238> [Accessed 18 December 2011].

Taylor, D. B. 2011a. Beginning the writing process, *WRT300: Writing in Health Sciences.* University of Toronto, unpublished.

Taylor, D. B., 2011b. Using sources and avoiding plagiarism, *WRT300: Writing in Health Sciences.* University of Toronto, unpublished.

Taylor, D. B., 2013. *Writing skills for nursing and midwifery students.* London: Sage.

Tourangeau, A. E. et al., 2007. Impact of hospital nursing care on 30-day mortality for acute medical patients. *Journal of Advanced Nursing,* 57(1), pp. 32–44.

U.S. Department of Health and Human Services, National Institutes of Health, National Centre for Complementary and Alternative Medicine, 2011. *Yoga for health: an introduction,* [pdf] Washington, DC: NCCAM. Available at: <http://nccam.nih.gov/health/yoga/introduction.htm> [Accessed 20 December 2011].

Waltz, C. F., Strickland, O. L. and Lenz, E. R., 1991. *Measurement in nursing research.* 2nd ed. Philadelphia: F. A. Davis.

Wolff, A.C., Ratner, P. A., Robinson, S. L., Oliffe, J. L. and McGillis Hall, L., 2010. Beyond generational differences: a literature review of the impact of relational diversity on nurses' attitudes and work. *Journal of Nursing Management,* [e-journal] 18, pp. 948–969. Available through: Scholars Portal database [Accessed 18 December 2011].

WHAT IS A LITERATURE REVIEW?

7

WHAT IS A LITERATURE REVIEW AND WHY IS IT IMPORTANT?

'Literature' in the context of scholarly and scientific research does not refer to novels or other forms of creative writing. In the health professions, when we speak of the literature, we mean everything that has been written on a health topic by accredited scholars and researchers.

A 'literature review' or 'critical review' is a classification and evaluation of the literature, organized according to a guiding concept or topic. This could be a research question, a search for the best evidence-based practice, or an understanding of a problem/ issue within health. 'Critical' in this sense does not mean seeking out the negative; it means to evaluate something based on both its strengths and weaknesses and come to conclusions about its usefulness for understanding or solving the problem at hand.

Literature review tells us both what has and what hasn't been accomplished in an area of study. Think of scientific progress and our understanding of the human experience as stretching on a time line from prehistory to the stars. Literature review shows us where we are on the line – what we know (or think we know) and what we still hope to discover.

The ability to review the literature critically is important for a number of reasons. First, to become an expert in any field of endeavour, you must comprehensively know your field. Literature review develops two crucial skills which develop that knowledge:

- the ability to find the literature on a topic, and
- the ability to read, understand and evaluate it.

Researchers conduct reviews of the literature to justify proposed studies, to uncover patterns of findings in the field, to enter into scientific or professional debate, and to discover gaps in knowledge that lead to future research questions. Research reviews are often the first step toward making scientific discoveries and social interventions in our society.

In addition, critical reviews of state-of-the-art literature permit the health professional to make informed decisions, to practise in an expert manner, and to influence policy in his or her field. We should make a distinction here between making a decision and solving a problem. Problem-solving refers to situations in which there is one right answer that can be determined and applied; in contrast, decision-making involves tradeoffs among alternatives. Critical review helps us weigh the available alternatives and synthesize them into best practice or policy.

Finally, in course assignments, literature review helps you demonstrate knowledge of the field of study of the course. It demonstrates your ability to find relevant published material and to evaluate what you find.

To conclude, a good literature review is not just a summary, but a critical evaluation and synthesis. The best critical appraisals are:

1 organized around and directly related to the topic they explore;
2 a summary of what is and is *not* known about the topic within the literature;
3 able to identify areas of controversy and problem;
4 able to identify future directions for research, practice, policy, or theory.

Questions to ask yourself about your review of literature

1 Do I have a specific topic, problem, or research question which my literature review helps to define?
2 What type of literature review am I conducting? Am I looking at issues of theory? methodology? policy? quantitative

research (e.g., studies of a pathiophysiological process)? qualitative research (e.g., studies of loneliness among rural single mothers)?

3   What is the scope of my literature review? What types of publications am I using (e.g., journals, books, government documents, popular media)? What disciplinary databases am I searching? (e.g., nursing, medicine, psychology, sociology)?

4   How good are my information-seeking skills? Has my search been wide enough to ensure I've found all the relevant material? Has it been narrow enough to exclude irrelevant material? Is the number of sources I've used appropriate for the length of my paper?

5   Is there a specific relationship between the literature I've chosen to review and the problem I've formulated?

6   Have I critically analyzed the literature I use? Do I just list and summarize authors and articles, or do I assess them? Do I discuss the strengths and weaknesses of the material I cite?

7   Have I cited and discussed studies contrary to my perspective?

8   Will the reader find my literature review relevant, appropriate, and useful?

Questions to ask yourself about each book or article you're reviewing

1   Has the author formulated a problem/issue?

2   Is the problem/issue ambiguous or clearly articulated? Is its significance (scope, severity, relevance) discussed?

3   What are the strengths and limitations of the way the author has formulated the problem or issue?

4   Could the problem have been approached more effectively from another perspective?

5   What is the author's research orientation (e.g., interpretive, critical science, combination)?

6   What is the author's theoretical framework (e.g., psychoanalytic, developmental, feminist)?

7   What is the relationship between the theoretical and research perspectives?

8   Has the author evaluated the literature relevant to the problem/issue? Does the author include literature taking positions s/he does not agree with?

9   In a scientific research study, how good are the three basic components of the study design (i.e., population, intervention, outcome)? How accurate and valid are the measurements? Is the analysis of the data accurate and relevant to the research question? Are the conclusions validly based upon the data and analysis?

10 In popular literature, does the author use appeals to emotion, one-sided examples, rhetorically-charged language and tone? Is the author objective, or is s/he merely 'proving' what s/he already believes?

11 How does the author structure his or her argument? Can you 'deconstruct' the flow of the argument to analyze if/where it breaks down?

12 Is this a book or article that contributes to our understanding of the problem under study, and in what ways is it useful for theory or practice? What are its strengths and limitations?

13 How does this book or article fit into the topic or research question I am exploring?

TYPES OF LITERATURE REVIEW

There are many categories of literature review, and numerous (often synonymous) names used to describe them. They range in scope from a review of a single article to meta-reviews covering thousands of research studies. Here is a list of the most common general names for literature review you are likely to encounter:

Critique or systematic critique

Critical appraisal

Critical evaluation

Critical review

Literature summary

Literature survey

Literature synthesis

Review

Review of the literature

Some names, however, refer to specific forms of literature review:

Annotated bibliography: also called a 'critical bibliography' or just a 'bibliography.'

A set of entries, each of which identifies, briefly summarizes, and critically evaluates a study, article, or book. Described below.

Book review: a critical review of a single book, usually one that has been recently published. Described below.

Comparative review: summary, evaluation and comparison of two or three research studies. Also called 'summary and critique'.

Comprehensive review: a requirement for thesis and dissertation writing; it will form an entire chapter (occasionally two) of a thesis or dissertation. Described below.

Conceptual review: also called a 'conceptual literature review' or a 'theoretical review', this reviews articles and/or books about theories, conceptual frameworks and models. This type of literature plays a crucial role in patient/family-centred care, qualitative research, nursing history and theory, and other areas.

Evidence-based practice report: identifies and evaluates all the literature on a practice-based question in order to determine what is the best available research evidence on which to base practice. Described below.

Review article: an article in a journal or a scholarly database that synthesizes all the literature on a topic in order to evaluate its overall strength and make recommendations for future research. These are helpful sources when you are looking for titles of scholarly articles to consult.

Peer review: a review by an expert on the topic of an article that has been submitted for publication, as part of the acceptance process. The expert will recommend acceptance, acceptance with revision, or rejection.

Summary and critique: a short paper that consists of a brief section of summary followed by a longer section of critique. A summary and critique may review only one study or article, or may compare two-three. Globally, this is probably the most common literature review assignment in health sciences programs. The purpose may be to answer an assigned question or one that you develop (perhaps a PICO question). Or the purpose may be just to come to a conclusion about the quality and usefulness of the article[s]. Described in detail below.

Systematic review: this is the term for a literature review that is focused on a single research question and tries to identify, evaluate and synthesize all the high quality research evidence relevant to the question. Many use a technique called 'meta-analysis', which is a statistical method of combining evidence. It has become essential for all professionals involved in the delivery of health care to know how to read and apply systematic reviews. A primary goal of a systematic review is to minimize bias, but critiques of systematic reviews find that they are not always reliable and lack a universally agreed upon set of standards and guidelines. Nonetheless, they are extremely helpful sources. Perhaps the most widely used source of systematic reviews is *The Cochrane Database of Systematic Reviews.*

Annotated (critical) bibliography

An annotated bibliography (also called a critical bibliography or just a bibliography):

- Is a set of individual entries, as short as a reference citation plus a couple of sentences, or as long as a page. Each entry identifies, briefly summarizes, and briefly evaluates a study or article.
- Usually has an overall introduction to state the scope of coverage and formulate the question, issue, or concept the material illuminates.
- Usually has an overall conclusion to sum up the overall quality of the articles and what they contribute as a whole to our understanding of the topic.

A critical bibliography provides the reader with the following information about each article or book:

- The full bibliographic information in proper APA or Harvard reference style.
- A summary of the contents. Be very brief – less than half your entry. In the case of a research study, your reader wants to know:
    o   the researchers' purpose or question;
    o   the type of study;
    o   what they did;
    o   what they found;
    o   what they concluded.
- A brief description of the strengths, weaknesses, and usefulness of the article/book.

Use wording that is as precise as possible – with such limitations in length, you can afford no wasted words. But you must also be self-contained and give readers everything they need to know. For example, you can't ask them to go elsewhere to understand what an abbreviation stands for, so you need to spell it out in full the first time you use it (except the generally known ones like UN, WHO, HIV/AIDS). Finally, you need to be informative. It's a good idea, after you finish an entry, to set it aside for a couple of days. Then read it, pretending you've never read the original article, and ask yourself two questions: am I getting everything I need to know to understand the overall content of this article, and am I getting a sense of its overall quality and usefulness?

Summary and critique

Sometimes you may be assigned a study to summarize and critique; at other times, you may be asked to search the literature and choose a relevant study yourself. Summary and critique writing is an important skill – all health professionals need the ability to capture essential information and ideas, analyze them, and communicate that analysis clearly.

As its name says, this form of review has two sections, a summary and a critique. The summary is always shorter than the critique, generally not more than a quarter of the total length. Summary and critique assignments are generally anywhere from one to five pages long. A reader who has no prior knowledge of the research you are reviewing should come away from your summary and critique with a clear sense of its contents and usefulness.

A summary is a short description of an article (or sometimes a book) that highlights its main points and information. A critique is a 'careful examination of all aspects of a study to judge its strengths, limitations, meaning, and significance' (Burns & Grove, 1995, p. 545). The descriptions in Chapter 8 of the structure and content of quantitative and qualitative research articles will help you identify the strengths and weaknesses of research.

Reporting verbs: some of the verbs you use will indicate to the reader that you are describing the research and others indicate your evaluation of it:

Verbs that describe neutrally

study	do	analyze
find	carried out	point out
state	explain	focus
claim	propose	develop
say	discuss	observe
argue	describe	expand
conclude	note	replicate
conduct	report	

Verbs that suggest strength

show

demonstrate

reveal

establish

establish conclusively

Verbs that suggest strength but not conclusivity

suggest

indicate

attempt

Verbs that suggest weakness

fail to show/demonstrate/establish

omit

Comparing research studies

Broadly speaking, there are two ways to organize a comparison paper. The first common structure is to discuss one study, then the other, then conclude with a synthesis section. The synthesis (from the Greek -*syn*, to bring together) brings together the key points you have made about similarities and differences. It also sums up your judgment on how the quality and usefulness of the two studies compare:

FIRST OPTION

Section One: Study A summary and critique

Background and research problem/questions

Methodology (study design, sample, intervention, measurements)

Results

Discussion/conclusions

Summary evaluation of Study A's quality and usefulness

Section Two: Study B summary and critique

Background and research problem/questions

Methodology (study design, sample, intervention, measurements)

Results

Discussion/conclusions

Summary evaluation of Study A's quality and usefulness

Section Three: Synthesis of Studies A & B

Comparative critique of background/research problems/questions

Comparative critique of methodologies

Comparative critique of results

Comparative critique of discussions/conclusions

Concluding comparison of quality and usefulness

The other common option for a comparative review is to organize it as a series of topic comparisons, like this:

SECOND OPTION

Section One: Background/aims/questions: comparative summary and critique of A & B

Section Two: Methodologies: comparative summary and critique of A & B

Section Three: Results: comparative summary and critique of A & B

Section Four: Discussions/conclusions: comparative summary and critique of A & B

Section Five: Synthesizing summary of A & B's strengths and weaknesses and concluding comparison of quality and usefulness

Book reviews

A book review uses a summary and critique structure that is similar to what we have seen in the other forms of literature review:

- full bibliographic information in a header;
- who the author is and her or his credentials/appropriateness for writing this book;
- who the book is written for/who would be most interested in this book;
- summary of the contents followed by a critique of the contents;
- *or* summary and critique of the contents organized according to the sections of the book;
- final evaluation of its quality and usefulness to its audience

Books differ from articles in a number of important ways, but probably the most obvious one is length. Books can take much wider perspectives on a topic than any article could, and delve much deeper. Another feature is that the 'voice' of the writer(s) is much stronger because it has so much longer to develop and persuade. For this reason, book reviews should include a discussion of who wrote the book.

Perspective and bias

There is no such thing as a totally objective writer. Everyone who writes has particular interests and life experiences that influence the angle, or 'point of view', from which he or she approaches a topic. We call this a 'perspective'. Perhaps it is:

- a particular theoretical framework or model (e.g., a feminist model applied to issues of gender inequity in obstetrical training), or
- a rhetorical purpose (e.g., a desire to persuade members of the general public to improve their health behaviours), or
- an experience-based practical perspective (e.g., the belief that one approach to pain management in burn cases is more effective than another).

The words 'perspective' and 'bias' have similar dictionary meanings in the *Longman Dictionary of Contemporary English*:

Perspective: 'a way of thinking about something, especially one which is influenced by the type of person you are or by your experiences.'

http://www.ldoceonline.com/dictionary/perspective

Bias: 'an opinion about whether a person, group, or idea is good or bad which influences how you deal with it.'

http://www.ldoceonline.com/dictionary/bias_1

Nonetheless, we consider a bias to be a negative, conveying a sense that something is being hidden, or as exerting an unreasonable or even unethical influence. As you write, you should try to be conscious of these two frames of reference:

1   The framework and perspective of the author of the book. In the case of an edited book, there is another level: the framework and perspective of the book's editor.
2   Your own framework and perspective on the topic.

Questions to ask about

Fundamentals

- Who is the audience this book is written for?
- What are the issues being addressed? Are they clearly formulated? Is the significance (scope, severity, relevance) discussed?

- What and how useful is the organization of the book?
- Is the book well or poorly written?
- What is the author's perspective or bias?
- If relevant, what is the author's research perspective?
- If relevant, what is the author's theoretical framework?

Methodology

- How does the rhetoric/language address the particular audience of the book?
- What are the strengths and weaknesses of the arguments?
- What kinds of evidence are used to support the arguments, and how is evidence used? Are there alternative ways of arguing from the same material?
- How would you counter or support the arguments?

Application

- What is the most effective application of the book?
- What further issues are raised as a result of the book?
- How does the book relate to the overall concerns of your topic or patients or your profession?
- In what ways is the book useful for the theory or practice of your field?

Evidence-based practice reports

In 1991, Gordon Guyatt, one of a group of doctors working at McMaster University's school of medicine in Canada, coined the phrase 'evidence-based medicine' to describe medical diagnoses based on the best research and clinical evidence available (Van Rijn, 2007). Like many great breakthroughs, it seems an obvious approach once someone has thought of it. But until the approach was developed, health professionals relied on past practice and consensus; further, new practices took a great deal of time to spread and become universally adopted. Evidence-based medicine, and by extension evidence-based practice, is based on the principle that evidence takes precedence over consensus. As Dr. Brian Haynes, chair of the department of clinical epidemiology and biostatistics at McMaster said, it 'is an attempt to ensure that the evidence is coming from research that is properly valued – not overvalued or undervalued – and that that evidence doesn't have to wait 20 years for implementation' (Van Rijn, 2007).

With Dr David Sackett, Guyatt developed what is still the most widely used system for ranking the evidence produced by research into five levels of strength.

An evidence-based report is structured in sections that do the following:

- define the problem and its significance;
- describe the literature search for the evidence;

- describe the process of selecting the best evidence;
- weigh the evidence and make a recommendation for practice.

There is more detail on writing an evidence-based report in the forthcoming companion to this book, *Advanced Writing Skills for Nursing and Midwifery Students*.

Comprehensive reviews

Types of comprehensive review: Review article, systematic reviews (Cochrane database, etc.), meta-analyses, dissertation chapters.

A comprehensive review systematically overviews, summarizes, and critiques the current state of knowledge about a specific topic. A comprehensive review of research studies also includes a discussion of methodological issues and suggestions for future research. Readers want more than just a descriptive list of articles and books. It is usually a bad sign when every paragraph of a review begins with the names of researchers. Instead, reviews should be organized into useful, informative sections that present themes or identify trends.

The introduction of a review is typically short. Its purpose is to tell the reader how the review is organized. The body may provide an overview of weaker studies or studies that share similar methods, followed by greater individual attention to important studies. Or, more likely, it may be divided into sections (usually with headings) that cover important areas, providing comparable information about each study. There are numerous ways to organize the sections, for example, studies can be grouped according to:

- theoretical premises;
- related independent variables (see Chapter 8);
- related dependent variables (see Chapter 8);
- type and strength of design, such as uncontrolled case studies up to randomized control trials;
- findings.

The final component of the review is an overall summary and critique, summarizing the overall strengths and weaknesses of the body of literature and suggesting future directions for the literature. In long reviews, the individual subsections of the body will also conclude with a brief summary.

In the final year of many nursing programs, students are asked, as a dissertation, to design a research question and conduct a comprehensive review that is as long as 10,000–12,000 words. For these students, there is a much longer discussion on how to design a research question and write a comprehensive review in the forthcoming companion to this book, *Advanced Writing Skills for Nursing and Midwifery Students*.

- Two final, small notes on grammar and usage:

1 'research' is a non-count noun and therefore has no plural form. We might say 'a large body of research' or 'research

was conducted', but not 'many researches were conducted'. The word 'study', however, has both singular and plural forms: 'a study was conducted' or 'five studies were conducted'.

2   'conducted' is preferred to 'done' in scientific writing when describing research.

FURTHER READING

Burns, N. & Grove, S. K. (195). *Understanding nursing research*. Philadelphia. PA: W. B. Saunders.

HOW TO REVIEW THE LITERATURE

8

OVERVIEW

- Evaluating quantitative (QN) and qualitative (QL) research
- The parts of a quantitative research article and what to look for
- The parts of a qualitative research article and what to look for
- Further reading

This chapter has two objectives:

1 to help you become familiar with the types of research most common in the nursing literature and related bodies of literature (primarily medicine, psychology and sociology);
2 to give you a variety of checklists and questions to guide your critical appraisal of the different types of research.

EVALUATING QUANTITATIVE (QN) AND QUALITATIVE (QL) RESEARCH

To critique research, we first need to understand what it is. Research is 'a systematic investigation to establish facts, principles or generalizable knowledge'. [You can find this definition at: section 1.1(d), www.sshrc.ca/English/programinfo/policies/index. htm.] When we critique a study, we examine the system the researchers use (called its 'design'); the methods they use; how they analyze what they find; and the facts, principles or knowledge they claim to have established.

There are two broad categories of research, quantitative and qualitative (also called traditional and interpretative). These are abbreviated here as QN and QL. Increasingly, researchers conduct studies (called 'mixed methods' studies) that combine the two. For example, someone who is studying nursing issues in neuroscience and trauma might investigate a particular cognitive consequence of traumatic brain injury, but also interview patients about the impact it has had on their ability to conduct their daily lives.

- Quantitative research designs
  - experimental and quasi-experimental
  - correlational
  - observational
  - case study
  - survey
  - developmental
- Qualitative research designs
  - ethnography
  - hermeneutics
  - phenomenology
  - grounded theory
  - narrative
  - arts-based
  - action

Quantitative research uses the scientific method to discover knowledge of the body as a diseased versus an undiseased organism. In this fundamental way it differs from qualitative research, which seeks knowledge of the body as a lived experience, and seeks to understand the social, psychological and behavioural aspects of health and health care. The purpose of QN research is to arrive at an understanding of the world by describing and explaining phenomena through established principles for scientific research. What, it asks, causes disease in the body? What can we apply to the diseased body so that the effect is a restoration of the undiseased body? QN research is hypothesis-driven; in other words, researchers predict what will happen if they conduct a test or experiment in a controlled setting. Then they conduct their research and conclude whether the results support (or don't) their prediction.

QN research breaks down situations it seeks to study into key aspects called 'variables', which simply means the thing the researchers are going to change (called the independent variable) and the things they hope will change as a result (called the dependent variables). In medical and nursing research, the independent variable is often referred to as a 'risk factor'. The researchers perform a treatment or procedure that manipulates the independent variable in some way[s], observe and record what happens to the dependent variables, and then measure and statistically analyze these results (also called 'findings') in order to draw their conclusions. For example, researchers might hypothesize that the independent variable of yoga has an influence (called a 'correlation') on the dependent variable of stress among pregnant women.

They will then perform a study on two equivalent groups of pregnant women: first they measure the 'baseline' levels of stress in both groups. Then one group (the 'experimental' or 'intervention' group) receives a 'dose' of yoga classes over a certain period of time; the other (called the 'control' group) does not. Then they repeat the stress measurements and compare the dependent variable of stress between the two groups to see if there is any correlation to yoga, i.e., if the yoga has influenced a greater change in stress levels than no yoga.

We said earlier that QN research studies the diseased body, while QL research seeks knowledge of the body as a lived experience, or the 'lived body'. Qualitative studies seek an in-depth understanding of human behaviour (*how* we behave) and the reasons for it (why we make our decisions to behave certain ways). They explore how we experience both health and illness, and the many factors outside the pathophysiological process which impact that experience, such as our family and social supports, our socioeconomic level and educational background, our cultural/racial identities, and other social determinants of health. These are all variables within our lives that cannot be controlled in the same way that QN researchers control their variables. QN research collects data in numeric form and manipulates it statistically. QL research collects data in words and images, then teases out its meaning in a variety of analytical ways. Thus, qualitative researchers identify and formulate research topics from different perspectives and use very different methods of collection and analysis than quantitative researchers.

A final and very important difference between the two lies in their assumptions about the role of the researcher. In QN research, the researcher attempts to be an objective observer and to control or remove any impact (or 'bias') he or she might exert on the research process. In QL research, however, the assumption is that the best way to learn about a situation is to participate in it. Thus, the researcher is acknowledged as an active participant in the research process, sometimes in active collaboration with the participants.

Both types of research are important, and each has its drawbacks. With its reliance on fixed methods of collecting data, such as scales and questionnaires, quantitative research captures only the data that fits those pre-set limits and thus may misrepresent the complexities of the disease/illness process. Qualitative research, on the other hand, sometimes focuses too closely on individual results derived from small samples and is not easily used to make connections to larger groups of people or situations. As well, because the researcher plays an active role in the research, there is always the risk that the researcher's individual beliefs and values may overinfluence his or her data collection and analysis.

THE PARTS OF A QUANTITATIVE RESEARCH ARTICLE AND WHAT TO LOOK FOR

IMRAD or IMRD are the common abbreviations for the standard sections within published research studies: Introduction, Methods, Results, (Analysis), Discussion. Quantitative research strives for 'rigour'. A rigourously conducted study:

- has a tightly controlled design;
- uses methods that can be verified and repeated by other scientists;
- has precise measurement tools; and
- studies a sample that accurately represents the larger population of interest, so that the study results can be 'generalized' to the whole population.

What follows is a description of the sections you can expect to find in an article reporting on a quantitative study, although you will encounter variations of this structure. There are also questions and comments to guide you in judging the strengths and weaknesses of these studies as you critique them.

Title

A good title summarizes, as specifically as possible, what the study is researching. Does it do that? For example, 'Pain management for Wales' ageing population' is far less informative than 'Pain management techniques for chronic arthritis in five long-term care settings in Wales.'

Authors and their affiliations

Who are the authors of the study? What institutions and/or universities are they affiliated with? Does it seem to you that their qualifications and affiliations make them suitable people to be studying the topic? You can also look up or link to other articles they've written; that will give you a sense of their experience in their area of expertise. Looking briefly at their other work will also help you understand their current study more easily, as researchers frequently work on related topics over a number of studies.

Abstract

An abstract is a brief summary which condenses in itself the argument and all the essential information of a paper. You don't need to comment on the abstract in your critique, but reading the abstract gives you a good overall understanding of the article and makes it easier to follow.

Introduction

Background: The first thing the authors do is give background on the problem they are studying. For example, in a study on pain and chronic illness, the authors might outline the rising rates of chronic illness and the health risks of long-term use of common painkillers.

Significance and relevance of the problem: The authors should tell you who is affected by this problem and how. They should tell you why it is important that we solve it. What will happen if it isn't resolved? What if it is?

Statement of the purpose: The purpose of a study is generated from the problem. It tells us in a clear, concise statement what the specific goal or aim of the study is to address or study the problem.

Brief literature review: It is important for researchers to position their research on the timeline of our knowledge about the problem. In order for us to understand the need for their research, they need to give us a clear and concise summary of what previous research has and has not established, what its strengths and limitations are, and what the gap is that the current study seeks to fill.

Research purpose, aims, goals, objectives, questions, and/or hypotheses

Researchers will include some (but not likely all) of these. Although different in some important ways, they all have the same intent, which is to make clear, concise statements that identify and describe the reasons for conducting the study, what exactly it will study, and how the researchers are going to study it.

A research purpose, goal or aim identifies and describes the change to the problem the researchers hope will result from their study. For example, a study might have the following aim:

> To evaluate the nutrient intake of Finnish pregnant women and relate it to the use of vitamin/mineral supplements.

A research objective is more specific: it identifies and describes the independent and dependent variables that will be studied to address the problem. For example, an objective might be:

> To measure nutrient intake adequacy of vitamin/mineral supplement users and non-users among Finnish pregnant women.

More specific still, a research question is an interrogative statement that the researchers develop to direct their study. For example:

> What is the nutrient intake adequacy of Finnish pregnant women who use vitamin/mineral supplements compared to non-users?

Method

Study design: This refers to the method the authors use to carry out their study. Broadly speaking, there are two types of design in quantitative research: experimental and descriptive. In an experimental design, a treatment or intervention is given to one randomly selected group of participants and not given to another randomly selected group of participants (the 'control'). The control group has carefully defined characteristics that are equivalent to those of the treatment group. Researchers also control factors that go beyond the participants alone: they will establish controls to prevent any other variables from influencing the results – for example, they might exclude participants with medical conditions in addition to the one they are studying. This design, called a randomized control trial (RCT), is the most robust one for establishing cause-and-effect relationships, and it is considered the 'gold standard' of research designs.

Quasi-experimental designs do not randomize their participants into treatment and control groups. They are used when it isn't ethically possible to have a control group – for example, if you are studying a life-saving surgery, you cannot withhold the surgery from one group of patients. Or it may not be practically possible to have a control group, for example, when researchers want to assess whether some intervention that is currently being used has made a difference since it was first initiated. These researchers might use case histories and chart reviews rather than current patients in what is called a retrospective design. For example, if we want to know if a particular smoking cessation campaign instituted ten years ago has worked, we could look at lung cancer rates in a geographic area where the campaign took place compared to one where it didn't. But even if the rates are lower, we can't claim to have proved the campaign caused the effect of lower rates because we have no way of controlling variables that have occurred in the past. Nonetheless, quasi-experimental designs make a very important contribution by enhancing internal validity when randomization is not possible.

Whether experimental or quasi-experimental, the authors should describe the following aspects of their design:

- Do they identify independent, dependent and other research variables?
- Do the researchers identify extraneous or confounding variables? These are variables that could distort the effects of the independent variable or that cannot be controlled by the researchers (either because they weren't anticipated or because they emerged only after the study started).

Description of the sample and setting

'Sample' refers to the subset of the population that has been selected for study. For example, rather than studying all Finnish pregnant women, researchers will recruit a number of individuals whose demographic characteristics (age, socioeconomic status, education level, and others) make them representative of that larger population. 'Sampling' refers to the process of selecting the sample. Look for these things:

- Who was eligible to be included in their study (inclusion criteria) and who was not (exclusion criteria)?
- How and where did they find the people who were eligible, and is it clear why they found them that way?
- Did they give a letter or form to inform potential participants about the study and get their 'informed consent' to participate? Do they tell you their research was approved by an ethics review board or some other ethics approval process? Researchers have an ethical obligation to protect the

well-being of their participants; to do no harm; and to protect confidentiality and privacy. In other words, they should treat human participants as they would be treated, and treat animal subjects humanely.

- How large was their sample? Do they explain how they know that sample was large enough to produce usable results?
- How many participants are there at the beginning compared to the end? Do they account for any participants who left the study before it was completed (called 'sample mortality')?
- How many groups are there and how many in each group? The numbers should be equivalent – if they aren't, do the authors tell you why?
- If the balance of males and females among the participants seems important to you, based on what they are studying, do they make an attempt to balance the numbers?

The setting refers to where the study is conducted. Settings can be natural, partially controlled or highly controlled. It should be clear to you why they chose this setting, and how they controlled it (if they needed to).

Methods of measurement

Researchers should describe the 'instruments' they used to measure their study variables. These may be scales and questionnaires, physiologic measurements, and/or observations.

- Do they describe the instrument[s] they are using to measure their study variable? Do they say who developed it? If the authors developed it themselves, they should describe their development process.
- Do they describe how they know their instrument is both reliable and valid for measuring what it is supposed to measure? 'Reliability' refers to the extent to which it measures consistently. 'Validity' refers to the degree with which it measures accurately.

Data collection process

They will then describe how they performed the tests, measurements, etc., on the participants. If it was necessary for researchers or participants to be 'blind', they should describe how they did this. If the researchers themselves didn't collect the data, they should describe how those people were trained.

Results

Results sections describe what they found, that is, the data they collected. We expect to learn how the authors analyzed the data they collected and what results they obtained to answer their research questions.

Data analysis procedures

In quantitative research, statistical methods are used to analyze the data. Statistics can help to determine if the relationships between independent and dependent variables are due to chance or due to the effect of the treatment (i.e., cause and effect). Unless you have taken a course in statistics, you will find these sections hard to follow. The word to look for is 'significance'. Significance in this context does not have the common meaning of 'importance'. Instead, it is a specific term – a significant result is one that is unlikely to have occurred by chance.

Presentation of results

Results are presented in the same order as the research questions or hypotheses, and are given from most important to least important, or strongest to weakest. The text should give the important information, with tables and figures to provide full details.

Discussion

The purpose of this section is to interpret the results in order to answer their research question[s] or support the hypotheses. Discussion sections interpret the results to make points. For example, a results section might say:

> In the treatment group, 116 (84%) participants reported improvements in functional ability.

The discussion section might then say:

> The unexpectedly high percentage (84%) of participants who reported improvements in functional ability suggests that this pain management technique, although controversial, is highly effective in older adults with arthritis.

The section should discuss the results in the same order they were presented in the results section.

Relationship to previous literature

The argument of this sub-section runs as follows: (1) here are the ways in which our study is similar to previous studies – this supports what we found. (2) Here are the ways in which our results are different from previous studies: (a) either their study or ours was flawed, incomplete, or simply different in some way; (b) we've identified the causes of the differences and they don't matter. Finally, the authors argue that: (3) Our results advance our previous knowledge on the problem in these ways.

Identification of the limitations

No study is perfect – it isn't possible. So it's important for the authors who, after all, know their study best, to identify what the weaknesses in their study were. They will also identify any ways in which future studies could overcome or improve them.

Conclusions

This section completes the train of argument that ran from the results (here's what we found) to the discussion (here's the relationship between what we found and the question we asked) by adding conclusions (here's what we can conclude about our research problem and the larger population our results can be generalized to). The authors should also do the following:

Identification of implications for the field

The authors should describe any larger purposes for research, policy, theory or practice that this study contributes to. They need to convince us that their study has added to our current body of knowledge.

Recommendations for future research

This may be its own sub-section or be combined with a description of the study's strengths and limitations. They may suggest that future research make changes in methodology, or they may suggest new research questions or new populations for study.

References

Their references are an excellent resource for you, an easy way to discover what the current and important literature is on this research area. You will also get a sense of who the major researchers and theorists are as you read multiple articles and see the same sources cited in many of them.

Acknowledgments

Academic and scientific journals have ethics guidelines that require authors to acknowledge their funding sources and any possible conflicts of interest. For example, there has been a number of high-profile cases in which it was revealed that researchers had been funded by pharmaceutical companies to test their drugs, and then published results that were falsely positive or which omitted negative findings or side effects.

THE PARTS OF A QUALITATIVE RESEARCH ARTICLE AND WHAT TO LOOK FOR

Like QN research, QL also strives for 'rigour' but in different ways. It strives for 'trustworthiness' in interpretations of the data. One of the great challenges of qualitative research lies in finding a practical tool for assessing it. In an important article on evaluating qualitative health research, Eakin and Mykhalovskiy (2003) note that quantitative health research derives from the work of clinical epidemiologists in developing evidence-based medicine. For this reason, they argue, quantitative checklists like the one in the last section focus on *how* the research is conducted; that is, they focus on 'procedure'. As Eakin and Mykhalovskiy put it, quality is judged 'on the basis of the researcher having made the right choice of method and having executed it in the right way' (p. 190). As QL researchers attempt to capture in language the richness and fluidity of human life and health, however, their methods also need to be flexible and diverse. Their methods become resources for engaging with and understanding the topic of inquiry and their findings. These methods resist the standardization that makes quantitative research so much easier to checklist. Instead, Eakin and Mykhalovskiy advocate focusing our evaluative energy on the analytic content of the research, its 'substantive' offering, that is, what the authors actually say about the phenomena they have investigated and how they relate their research practices to their findings (p. 191).

Unfortunately, the dominant stream within health research was historically (and still remains) QN. In addition, the world of health care management is a very pragmatic place and QL research is often not generalizable to larger populations or intended to propose solutions to immediate problems. For these reasons and others that have to do with the publication process, the appraisal of QL research is usually done using templates derived from QN checklists. A good example of this is the widely used Critical Appraisal Skills Programme (CASP) checklist for qualitative studies (available at http://www.casp-uk.net/).

Because of the publication process, many QL researchers structure their articles and use language that is consistent with the widely-used checklists. Thus, the questions proposed below to help you evaluate QL studies draw from traditional checklists but also focus on the substantive aspects of QL research. The goal is a) to help you explore how the different elements of the research contribute to the authors' ability to derive meaning from their findings and b) to help you use the research to improve your practice and advocate for your patients.

Introductory material

- Do the authors introduce their study with the background, significance, and relevance of the topic they are studying?
- Do they identify a purpose for their study?

The research question

- Does the research question provide a 'positioning device' for understanding the nature of the investigation and its findings? Does it feel like a good starting point?
- Does it identify and describe the kinds of knowledge the researchers were seeking in/through the research process?
- If their research question[s] changed through the process of conducting the research, do the authors tell you how, when and why?

The researcher[s]

Unlike the objectivity and 'view from outside' that is expected of QN researchers, in QL the researchers are assumed to be subjective – otherwise they wouldn't be able to engage with their participants and develop a 'view from inside'. Thus, it's very important for them to tell us about some of the following things at least:

- Do the researchers tell you anything about themselves? Any personal background? How they came to be interested in researching this topic?
- Do they describe any aspects of their 'social location'? Social location refers to the position we occupy within our society. That position is determined by our gender, age, class, income, education, family and social network, among others. When researchers consider their social location, it helps both them and us to understand how all these factors will affect the way they engage with their research and the ways they interpret it. It's especially important if they are studying a society that is not the one they belong to. Unfortunately, it is generally the case that researchers in developed countries have greater resources for travelling to developing countries to conduct research than the opposite.
- Did they engage in any self-reflexive process? Do you get the sense that it allowed them to approach their research with creativity and sensitivity?
- Can you identify their theoretical or conceptual 'location'? In other words, what kinds of theory shape their perspective on their research topic?
- Do they talk about how their theoretical location shapes the way they analyze and interpret their results? They may also talk about how the act of conducting and analyzing their research altered the theoretical location they started from.
- In describing their personal, social and theoretical relationship with their research, researchers need to choose what elements to describe. Do you think what they describe helps you understand the role these elements played in their data collection and analysis?

Theoretical framework

Most qualitative research identifies the theoretical perspective that lies behind the research, although the authors may not always do so explicitly. Some theoretical perspectives are what we call 'macro' perspectives, that is, they address large domains about the way the world is and how people behave. You can understand the macro-perspective of a researcher by asking yourself:

- Are they studying how people **experience** something (e.g., a life event such as a birth or chronic illness). In philosophy, this is called **phenomenology**, the study of the structure of experience.
- Are they studying how people come to **know** things (e.g., from family, education, media, society at large) or what they consider **knowledge** (e.g., that immunization is safe or not safe for children) or how health knowledge is socially

created (e.g., by whether a community has a Western-style medical clinic or a healer practising traditional medicine). In philosophy, this is called **epistemology**, the study of what constitutes knowledge and how we know it.

- Are they studying issues central to our **being** as humans such as our moral and ethical being, or our relationship with death? In philosophy, this is called **ontology**, the study of the nature of being, existence, or reality.

Within macro-level theories, there are many 'middle-range' theories that allow researchers to use the abstract concepts of macro-level theories to help design research on specific social and health issues. Here are some of the major ones you are likely to encounter in the QL health literature:

Positivism: You may encounter discussion of positivism in QL research, but not as an approach that the researchers themselves are adopting. In the positivist approach, reality is seen as stable, fixed and measurable, and a 'right' explanation can be discovered for all phenomena if we search long and hard enough. This perspective lies at the heart of QN research, and is frequently criticized by QL researchers as inappropriate and not very useful for studying the complex, unpredictable behaviour of individuals and social groups.

Interpretative approaches: In opposition to positivism, QL researchers prefer to speak of the way we interpret reality, rather than about an objective reality.

Social constructionism: This approach sees reality as something that is socially constructed. For example, thanks in part to media, Western society equates thinness with health and moral goodness. It associates obesity, as measured by the BMI (Body Mass Index) with disease and moral failure. These theorists, however, would argue that 'obesity' is as much a social construction as it is a medical one, and that BMI, a measure originally developed within the insurance industry, is not only an inaccurate predictor of health status but it also has negative social and psychological consequences.

Critical theory approaches: Critical theory approaches focus on power inequities within society that are based on gender, class, race, and other social constructs.

Feminist approaches: Feminism, which was originally a movement devoted to gender issues and to achieving equality for women, has now expanded to consider intersecting issues that create power inequities. For example, although it is true globally that women experience inequity relative to men, the problems are worse for women of colour or women living in poverty or in developing countries that were previously colonized.

Participatory approaches: This approach sees research as co-constructed by researchers and participants, on the basis that although researchers are experts in the sense of formal academic training, the participants are the experts of their own lives and communities.

All theories are based on 'assumptions', that is, a belief that is used as the basis of an idea. For example, in the theoretical approaches given above, critical theory assumes that there are unequal power relationships in any society while the participatory approach assumes that people will work together collaboratively to achieve a common benefit.

Research design and methods

Here are the broad QL research approaches commonly used in the nursing literature:

Phenomenological (note: phenomenology is both a philosophy and a research method). The purpose of this research is to capture the 'lived experience' of participants. Their experiences are collected from a small number of participants through observation, interviews, video and audiotapes, and descriptions written by the participants. The researcher then examines the captured materials and attempts to describe them by staying as close to the 'phenomena' (the experiences) as possible. Phenomenological philosophy is used to describe and interpret the meanings the researcher derives from the data. When you read phenomenological research, ask yourself:

- Does the researcher attempt to stay close to the personal meaning described by the participant?
- Is the participant's 'voice' reflected in the interpretation or description?

Ethnographic: The aim of ethnography is to learn and understand cultural phenomena which reflect the knowledge and system of meanings within the life of a cultural group. Culture is defined in many ways, and as a term is sometimes applied very broadly, such as to an entire racialized group (sometimes offensively broad, as when people speak of 'Aboriginal' or 'Hispanic' culture, as though any statement about culture could be true when applied to so many individuals in and from so many places). Or the word can be applied as narrowly as to describe the group experience of nurses in a single labour/delivery unit.

One type of ethnographic research is called **community-based participatory research:** this research is conducted as an equal partnership between the formally trained researcher and the members of a community. The community and researcher collaborate at every stage, from deciding what problem to investigate, defining it, deciding on a research design, gathering resources, carrying out the research, interpreting the results, sharing the credit, and deciding how to put the results into action in the community. Ask yourself if you see this. If not, does the researcher tell you why? Or do you feel the researcher had unequal power in directing the research – if so, in what ways?

Grounded theory: grounded theory is related to phenomenological research in that it studies phenomena; for example, the stress and burnout experienced by newly graduated nurses. The intent of grounded theory as it was originally developed by Glaser and Strauss (1967) is to develop a theory that explains the phenomenon being studied. The name refers to the idea that the theory is 'grounded' in the data from which it emerges. In grounded theory, the researcher collects, organizes and analyzes data, and forms theory all at the same time. Data are collected from multiple sources and constantly compared with each other in order to code and categorize them into themes from which the theory is developed. Currently, however, it is not unusual for researchers to conduct a form of grounded theory research without necessarily developing a theory.

Historical: It is only by understanding where we have come from that we can truly understand who we are. For this reason, there is an ever-growing body of nursing research concerned with the history of nursing as a profession and the history of nursing knowledge. Unlike other forms of QL research, the 'participants' may no longer be living, so these researchers rely on historical 'artifacts', that is, documents, photos, journals, legal documents, historical archives, newspapers, and other forms of primary documentation that survive from the period under study and help the researcher build a picture of the values, beliefs and knowledge of society as it was. For example, through the historical evidence we have about Florence Nightingale's life, we can come to understand that it was her upper-class status – in the rigid class structure of Victorian England – which allowed her to advocate on the highest levels of government for the nursing profession. That allows us to make a comparison with the power structures of our own times and the challenges faced by nursing and midwifery around the world.

Whatever approach is used, the design of a QL study needs to be 'feasible'. By this we mean, is it doable? It should be practically feasible: ask yourself if the researcher has the personal qualities, life history, and training to gain access to and 'fit in' with the lives of the people or organizational culture being explored. Another part of practical feasibility involves resources, both of time and materials (including funding). Access is another issue, especially in studying groups with high mobility, such as homeless adolescents. It is especially important for the design to be ethically feasible, because QL research is often conducted with vulnerable populations.

Sample and setting: Samples are often small and focused. Settings are usually 'natural', meaning that participants are studied where they live or work. Alternatively, the participant and researcher may arrange to meet in a 'neutral' setting that is convenient for the participant. Ask yourself these questions:

- What information is provided about the characteristics of the participants or organizational setting? Does that information help you understand the interaction with the researcher and the data that were produced as a result?
- What information is provided about how the researcher recruited the participants? Why these particular participants? Did any of them decline to participate and if so, why? Do the researchers explain how they addressed ethical concerns? Do they describe any important ethical challenges in conducting research on this particular group of participants – for example, studying women in relationships where they are the victims of domestic violence might create safety issues for them. Did the researchers receive ethics approval from their own institution and any other appropriate organizations? Do they describe the process of getting informed consent from their participants? Do they persuade you that there were no risks to their participants from participating? Were there any benefits to their participants?
- Do you think the group of people or organizational setting is relevant to your own practice and patients? What do you feel you are learning from reading about them?

Generating and collecting data

- Do they describe how they generated or collected their data, and why they chose that method?
- If the researcher[s] modified the methods during the study (as frequently happens in qualitative research as part of the emergent design process), do they explain how this came about?
- Do they explain clearly what form the data were collected in (e.g., written documents such as surveys, researcher field notes, audio tapes, video)?
- How did they generate their data? Here are some common ways:
  o participant/non-participant observation;
  o field notes;
  o reflexive journals;
  o interviews;
  o focus groups and key informant interviews;
  o analysis of documents and other materials;
  o surveys and questionnaires.

Interviews: Interviews, with individuals or with groups (e.g., focus groups) are the most common source of data for QL health researchers. They are categorized as structured, semi-structured or in-depth. In a structured interview, the questions are carefully scripted, with every participant being asked exactly the same questions in the same order. For a semi-structured interview, the researcher designs a guide that sets an agenda for the interview, but allows the interviewees to speak to each item as they choose. In an in-depth interview, questions are 'open-ended'. They are designed to act as topic openers for the participant to take in any direction they like, and subsequent questions are then based on what the interviewee offers.

Interviews are a wonderful window into the inner world of participants, revealing what they think and feel about their lives and experiences. But interviews don't necessarily give a clear picture of how people behave, which may be very different from how they say in an interview that they behave.

Observational studies: Observational studies, as the name suggests, allow researchers to describe and understand what is going on in a particular social setting. They do not intervene to direct or control what happens, and the data they collect is the naturally occurring talk and behaviours of people's everyday lives and interactions.

Case studies: 'Case study' is a broad term, referring to the process of studying a phenomenon within its context (Green & Thorogood, 2004, p. 36). Case studies are used in both QN and QL research, and in fact were used in QN long before QL came along. In QL, 'case' may be applied widely – for example, funding of a women's HIV/AIDS support program (the phenomenon) and its impact within its context, in this case a historically poor neighbourhood in the capital city of Namibia, a country with one of the world's highest HIV/AIDS rates.

At the other end of the spectrum, the case that is studied may be a single person – a 'life history'. An example would be collecting the life story of a person who has been in and out of mental institutions and jail since his teens. There is great value in learning such a story, as it illuminates the failures within the mental health and judicial systems.

Nursing students are often asked to write a 'case study' as an assignment. This always includes a major element of life history and its role at all steps of the nursing care, including the care plan. But this type of case study also covers the medically-oriented dimensions of nursing care, including the pathophysiological process, diagnosis, and medical interventions. There is a sample case study paper in Chapter 12.

Surveys and questionnaires: The basic idea of a survey or questionnaire is the same whether a study is quantitative or qualitative: it is a means of collecting the same set of data from every 'case' in the study (Green & Thorogood, 2004, p. 36). In the case of QN research, however, the purpose is to narrowly control the responses so that the data collected can then be expressed in numeric form. A 'purely' qualitative survey, on the other hand, would use only open-ended questions. In actuality, a great many QL surveys and questionnaires use questions of both kinds, for example, collecting demographic data before offering a set of semi-structured or open-ended questions.

Data analysis

- Do they describe their findings clearly?
- Do they describe the process they went through to analyze their findings?
- Do they explain how they chose which data to analyze, and what they chose to omit?
- If they used a grounded theory approach, do they explain how they derived their categories/themes from their data? Does it seem to you that the themes that emerged in their analysis are reflected in their examples and quotations? Grounded theory methods that seek patterns (such as coding, concept mapping, emerging themes) should leave you with a feeling of rich description. They should also leave you with a clear sense of how the theoretical concepts the researcher began from have contributed to the analysis.
- How do they interpret their findings?
- If relevant, do they try to establish the following elements of their analysis? Remember, these concepts may not be relevant to all QL studies:
  o Rigour: the pursuit at all stages of a study of accuracy and precision.
  o Transferability: the extent to which the results can be transferred to a larger population. In QN research, this is called 'generalizability' and is established through statistical analysis. In QL, transferability is established by considering the kinds of relationships between the study sample and the larger group it represents.
  o Credibility: this is not an easy dimension to appraise, though its dictionary meaning is fairly straightforward:

'the quality of deserving to be believed and trusted' (LDCE). Those who are experienced in conducting and reading QL research are able to draw on their knowledge of previous studies; they also have background knowledge about the historical/social/political/theoretical contexts of the research. Nonetheless, students who are still learning these dimensions can ask themselves: 'Based on my appraisal of everything I've read in this study and about the researcher, do I feel convinced?'

o   Other terms you may encounter are 'dependability', 'confirmability', 'coherence', and 'authenticity'.

The narrative of a QL representation

We said above the QL is language-based, so you need to carefully consider the narrative of a study, that is, the story it tells. You also need to distinguish between the participant's narrative and the researcher's narrative. The former is that of the interviews; the latter is that of the researcher's interpretation or representation. The narrative dimension is especially relevant to ethnographic studies because they attempt to portray the concepts of physical and social health/illness in terms of people's lived experience:

- Is the writing richly detailed in describing both the facts about the participants and their feelings? Do you feel immersed in their lives?
- Is there a sense of the past and future of the participants, not just their present situation? Do you feel you are sharing in their life's journey?
- Does it touch you on an emotional level? Do you perhaps feel a connection between their lives and yours, or does the contrast help you understand your own life and practice in a new way?
- Is it an ethical narrative? That is, do you feel that there is mutual respect and sensitivity between the researcher[s] and participants?
- Does the narrative satisfy you rationally, so you feel convinced that the results mean what the authors say they do?

Conclusion: how valuable is the research?

- Do they consider how their research may be used? Do they discuss the contribution their study makes? It may be a contribution to the body of current research on the topic. It may contribute to practice, policy, or social and community action. It may contribute to our understanding of health within the context of social life.
- Do they identify new areas for research, or ways to continue their current research?

FURTHER READING

Burns, N., & Grove, S. K. (1995). *Understanding nursing research.* Philadelphia: W.B. Saunders.

Creswell, J. W. (2003). *Research design: Qualitative, quantitative, and mixed method approaches.* Thousand Oaks, CA: Sage Publications.

Critical Skills Appraisal Programme (CASP). *Making sense of evidence: CASP critical appraisal checklist for qualitative studies.* Available at http://www.casp-uk.net/

Denzin, N. K., & Lincoln, Y. S. (2011). *The Sage handbook of qualitative research* (4th ed.). Thousand Oaks, CA: Sage Publications.

Domholdt, E. A. (1993). *Physical therapy research: Principles and applications.* Philadelphia: W. B. Saunders.

Eakin, J. M., & Mykhalovskiy, E. (2003) Reframing the evaluation of qualitative health research. *Journal of Evaluation in Clinical Practice* 9(2), pp. 187–194.

Glaser, B. G. & Strauss, A. L. (1967) *The discovery of grounded theory: Strategies for qualitative research.* Chicago, IL: Aldine.

Goubil-Gambrell, P. (1992). A practitioner's guide to research methods. *Technical Communication.*

Green, J., & Thorogood, N. (2004) *Qualitative methods for health research.* London: Sage.

Highly recommended. This book is intended primarily for students/practitioners in nursing and allied professions 'in both developed and developing countries, with little previous experience of social science theory, who need to … use or conduct qualitative research' (p.xiv).

Neutens, J., & Robinson, L. (2001). *Research techniques for the health sciences* (3rd ed.). Toronto, ON: Benjamin Cummings.

AN INTRODUCTION TO PROFESSIONAL WRITING 9

ACADEMIC VERSUS PROFESSIONAL WRITING

In this chapter, we will look at a variety of important forms of professional writing. Before we do, let's clear up the differences (and similarities) between academic and professional writing:

Academic writing refers to the writing you do as part of a program of study. Programs in nursing, midwifery and other health professions ask students to engage, broadly speaking, in two forms of writing: writing that integrates theory, research and practice; and reflective writing.

Professional writing refers to the writing you do as a health professional in accordance with the standards of your profession's regulatory body.

Clinical or agency writing refers to the professional writing you do in the context of your practice setting.

A good question . . .

Why write the long, complicated documents of academic writing if I never use it in the workplace?

Academic writing develops transferable abilities:

- the ability to make decisions that are objective and informed;
- the ability to grasp and describe complex situations, analyze them, and clearly articulate conclusions and recommendations;
- the ability to describe and argue;
- the ability to achieve language 'correctness' and persuasiveness;
- the ability to use and document sources.

Academic writing also develops perspectives:

- on social issues;
- on self: becoming a reflective practitioner;
- on human behaviour and interaction.

Table 9.1 Comparison of academic and professional writing

	Academic writing	Professional writing
Who is the audience?	• Professors, often standing in for a professional audience • The academic community	• Colleagues in your own field • Multidisciplinary team • Agency administrators • Government and Regulatory bodies • Legal/justice system • Clients • General public
What will your audience do with what you've written?	• Assess your understanding of the theory and research as applied to practice and assign a grade • Assess your development as a reflective practitioner and assign a grade	Make decisions and take action on, for example: • Treatment/intervention • Policy • Behaviour change • Funding • Replicating or carrying forward from what you did in practice

Table 9.1   (Continued)

	Academic writing	*Professional writing*
What is the purpose of writing?	• To demonstrate comprehensive knowledge of theory and research • To develop critical reading/thinking/writing skills • To appraise and conduct research • To become a reflective practitioner	• To report • To record • To recommend • To shape and evaluate policy • To propose and evaluate programs
What is the writing process?	• Iterative (reading, brainstorming, outlining, drafting, revising) • Idea-driven • Deadline-driven	• Often linear (e.g., forms, documentation, reports, requests) • Event-driven • Deadline-driven

But there are also similarities between academic and professional writing:

- both need an appropriate balance of description and argument;
- both use conventionalized/standardized structures that need to be learned; they force you to be adaptable to 'templates'
- both use conventional language, a 'technical discourse' that needs to be learned; they make you think about the tone and diction expectations of your audience;
- both require decisions about what to include in the space available;
- both require decisions about what to emphasize and how to use language to indicate emphasis;
- both must be both grammatically 'correct' and persuasive;
- both of them value clear, concise, logical writing;
- for both, the needs of the audience are always the first consideration:
  o Who is my audience?
  o What do they already know and what do I need to tell them?
  o What will they do with what I've written?
  o How much will/won't they read?

NURSING AND MIDWIFERY PORTFOLIOS

Andy Young (2007) defines a portfolio this way: 'A portfolio is a record of your clinical and professional nursing skills supported by a body of evidence. It also serves as a record of your clinical experience and journey from novice to expert'.

Professional colleges and regulatory bodies generally require health professionals, especially nurses and midwives, to maintain ongoing portfolios that are periodically reviewed. In the UK, for example, the National Health Service requires nurses to maintain a Knowledge and Skills Framework (KSF), a clinical portfolio that is reviewed annually by their employers within the NHS. Portfolios are also an important marketing tool if you wish to advance in your current position or move to a new one. CVs or résumés (described below) are an essential part of a job search, but a portfolio adds a whole new dimension by providing physical evidence of your skills and abilities. Likewise, they add a new dimension to your development as a person and a professional, because they actualize (make real) your goals, and allow you both to reflect back and plan for the future.

Oermann (2002) describes two types of professional portfolios: best-work and growth and development. **Best-work portfolios** are designed to be reviewed by others; they provide documented evidence of competencies and skills that are used by others to evaluate nurses for annual review, promotion and accreditation processes. 'Competencies' are specific and observable knowledge, skills and behaviours that are associated with effective functioning in a job. **Growth and development portfolios** allow nurses and midwives to monitor their own progress in meeting personal and professional learning goals; they are not intended for review by others, but materials from them are selected for inclusion in best-work portfolios.

Worldwide, portfolios are increasingly required as an assessment tool within nursing and midwifery programs. This is because a portfolio has the unique ability to capture learning over time in a way that tests or grades may not. It is a great advantage if you are required to build a portfolio during your student program, as that builds the skill and the habit of working on it, and gives you the opportunity for ongoing feedback. All you have to do, then, when you enter your post-registration career, is maintain the habit.

Guides on building and maintaining a portfolio often admonish people to work on theirs on a continuous basis, and to avoid the shoebox stuffed with documents and other artifacts. Or, as I call it (because I too am guilty of it), the archaeological system of filing. This 'system' can indeed work badly, as important documents have a habit of hiding themselves at exactly the moment you must put your hand on them. So, yes, it is always best to be proactive in maintaining your portfolio.

But life doesn't always allow us to be proactive, and as you enter your new career you will have an enormous lot of stuff thrown at you. As long as the 'shoebox' is actually an accordion folder that you have tabbed with the names of the parts of your portfolio, you'll be fine. It's easy to be proactive about tossing something into an accordion folder, and the work of seconds to jot down a few notes, on the front or back, about its relevance or meaning. The same is true for capturing reflective moments. Sometimes people will say they are too busy to be reflective, but in fact humans are by nature reflective beings. We think – sometimes obsess – over things that happen to us and what they mean to our lives. So when something about your day gets you thinking, and talking to your friends and family about it, why not also take a few minutes to write down what happened and what you are thinking/feeling right now? Into the folder (or your electronic portfolio folder) it goes, under 'reflective'. The more you put into your folder, the more material you have to work with. No need to decide now if something will be useful or not – just get it all in there. At this point, you are going for quantity. When you have a reason to fully update your portfolio – for accreditation or a new position – you are all set to sit down and work through the parts to update them using the folder materials. Your important materials won't have gone missing, and you'll have more than enough evidence to support them.

Although you are going for quantity, don't feel that because you've assembled a thick folder of evidence that you have to use it all. The folder is there as a resource to draw on as your portfolio changes over time.

Increasingly, both student and professional portfolios are created, maintained, and ultimately submitted online as e-portfolios. Much of what you collect, then, will already be in digital format, for example, photos, videos, scanned documents. The same principle as the physical accordion file holds true – whatever technology you use, maintain a portfolio folder on your central computer with files for the individual parts.

Formatting your portfolio

For a paper-based portfolio, use a three-ring binder. Use a tabbed divider for each section, even if there is only one sheet in the section. Each section gets a cover sheet listing the contents of the section (this is in addition to the listing in the portfolio's general Table of Contents). Include a cover sheet even if there is only one sheet in the section. Place each cover sheet and artifact into its own clear plastic page protector.

If you are building an e-portfolio, your program may provide an e-portfolio template, or there are numerous ones available online. Keep your e-portfolio backed up on a USB memory stick.

What to include in a portfolio

In general, every section of a portfolio should contain:

- descriptions of the relevant elements of your student and professional life;
- evidence, called 'artifacts', that support your descriptions;
- reflections on your artifacts and the personal/professional journey they represent.

An artifact is a physical record of an event – we might think of them as souvenirs of a trip. Like a souvenir photograph, a good artifact captures both the content and meaning of the event. For example, a care plan can be included not only to document your actions but also to allow you to reflect on how well you performed in a complex situation. An artifact may be a document such as a transcript of grades, a license, or a certificate. It may be a photograph. It may be job related, such as a job description, reference, list of previous employers, performance review forms, or record of committees you have belonged to. It may be a digital artifact such as a PowerPoint presentation or a poster. It may be creative work such as poetry, stories, or drawings that represent artistically the experience of you and/or your patients/families. In short, an artifact is almost anything that you think is relevant to your career and that will help you identify your achievements, skills and goals.

The names and content of the sections of your portfolio will vary depending on who is asking you for it:

- When it is a requirement within a nursing or midwifery program, it is to be hoped – but isn't always the case – that you are given a 'template' your instructors want you to follow. If you are given a template, it may be highly structured or it may allow considerable creativity on your part. You may be asked to maintain and submit your portfolio in traditional paper format, or you may be encouraged (even required) to submit it electronically.
- Institutions may require periodic submission of your portfolio in order to review your performance to date and potential for development. They often specify a particular format.
- Regulatory bodies may also require periodic submission of your portfolio for accreditation purposes, and often require a particular format, sometimes supplying electronic record sheets for you to follow.
- A job advertisement will ask for your CV or résumé as part of the application rather than your full portfolio. Even if not asked for, though, you may wish to bring your portfolio to the interview in case there is an opportunity to present it. When using a portfolio as part of an application for a job, make sure you include materials that demonstrate your skills are tailored to the needs of that particular organization. Similarly, include materials that demonstrate your abilities to fulfil the particular position you are applying for.

Whatever the format you use, it will include the following content sections or equivalents of them:

- a personal information sheet that lists your name and contact information, which should include your address, email address (if you have an institutional address, use that rather than your personal account), website (if you have one, but *not* your Facebook or other social media address), and telephone/mobile/cellphone; when you have graduated and successfully passed your licensure examinations, you will add your registration number[s].
- an up-to-date copy of CV (curriculum vitae) or résumé – see below;
- personal history;
- educational achievements and goals;
- practice history and goals;
- work in the community, volunteer or charity work: highlight your specific role in the organization and the skills you developed;

- reflection: a crucial component of any portfolio, reflection should occur within each of your sections and then have its own section that both sums up and expands on your other reflections.

To help you gather the points you want to make, think about the following questions:

Who am I? To plan for our futures, we need to understand our past and our present, that is, what has brought us to this point and where are we now in the journey of becoming or being a nurse/midwife. These questions will help you reflect on your life and where you are on your nursing/midwifery journey, as well as what details about it you want to offer:

- If I were asked to write one paragraph to tell the story of my life, what would I include?
- How would I describe my personality? What are the best and worst aspects of my character? What have been the 'defining moments' (the real highs and hows) of my personal life? In what way[s] did they change my approach to life?
- What have been the defining moments of my nursing/ midwifery journey to date?
- Who are the people who have had the greatest impact (positive and/or negative) on my life? On my nursing/ midwifery journey to date?
- What are my strengths and weaknesses as a practitioner?
- What do I have to offer a multidisciplinary team?
- What do I believe to be the biggest problems faced by nursing or midwifery today? These could be problems related to broader government policies, the structure of the healthcare system, the nursing/midwifery role, nursing/midwifery practice, etc.

For a student portfolio, these are some types of supporting evidence you could use:

- autobiographical story and/or a few vignettes (i.e., a brief written 'snapshot' of a defining moment in your life and what it meant);
- a description of your philosophy of nursing;
- a personal coat of arms you design to represent your nursing/ midwifery values and career goals;
- photos;
- short video.

My education:

- What has my education given me in terms of clinical/practice knowledge?
- What critical and analytic skills has my education given me?

- In what ways has my education contributed to making me a competent and reflective practitioner?
- What detailed examples from my education can I highlight and include in my portfolio to support my answer to those questions? A student portfolio could include:
  o successful course assignments (perhaps with the marker's feedback);
  o evidence of interprofessional education;
  o self-evaluations;
  o preceptor evaluations;
  o academic achievements, honours, awards and scholarships;
  o professional documents such as proof of education, licenses, and certifications (including renewal dates and hours completed toward recertification);
  o continuing education and professional development;
  o in-service education;
  o presentations and/or education sessions to colleagues, groups of patients, multidisciplinary teams, the community.

My clinical/practice experience: This can be organized according to your competencies and your cases.

- What are some specific examples of times I've applied the nursing process to direct and indirect care of my patients and their families?
- Do I practise evidence-based care?
- What are some examples of my ability to care sensitively for patients/families of diverse backgrounds?
- What do I do that promotes a nursing model of patient/family-centred care or a midwifery model of partnership and support for women's right to self-determination in life processes?
- What feedback (positive and negative) have I received from my preceptor, manager, colleagues, patients/carers/families?
- What do I consider my areas of greatest strengths and greatest challenges?
- Possible types of evidence:
  o descriptions of relevant, significant clinical experiences;
  o proof of acquired skills;
  o clinical journals that include current evidence-based research and reflection to improve patient care;
  o a course paper that describes the nursing process from assessment, diagnosis and medical/nursing interventions to nursing care plan and discharge planning guide;
  o cultural assessments;

- o   a concept map: a concept map is a way of graphically representing all dimensions of a patient's care, a concise web of information with a description of the patient at the centre; a concept map is a way of making sense, both in its details and its entirety, of all the patient information and the medical/nursing/midwifery process;
- o   health promotion/education projects you designed and implemented in the practice setting or community.

My work in the community: This section can highlight and provide examples of:

- health promotion/education projects;
- needs assessments;
- activist and advocacy efforts;
- collaborative community efforts;
- volunteer and charity work.

For reflection: how can I make a difference?

- What are my career goals?
- What are my practice goals?
- Do I hope to make a difference in the field of policy and social advocacy? In clinical expertise? In research? In nursing/midwifery care? In community health?
- What nursing and social theories are most relevant for me? How might I use them in my practice?
- What is my action plan for developing the skills and knowledge I will need?

For further reading

National Council for the Professional Development of Nursing and Midwifery. (2009, November). *Guidelines for portfolio development for nurses and midwives* (3rd ed.). Dublin: Author.

Oermann, M. H. (2002). Developing a professional portfolio in Nursing. *Orthopaedic Nursing, 21*(2), 73–78.

Young, Andy. (2007, January 1). Making your development portfolio work for you. *NursingTimes.net*. Retrieved from: http://www.nursingtimes.net/nursing-practice/student-nurses/making-your-development-portfolio-work-for-you/201130.article

CVS AND JOB APPLICATIONS
The curriculum vitae vs. the résumé

A curriculum vitae (literally, course of life) or résumé is always part of a job application. The *Gage Canadian Dictionary* gives these two terms as synonyms:

Curriculum vitae, résumé = summary of one's life, qualifications, etc. Résumé is the general term; curriculum vitae is used mainly in academic and professional situations.

Source: Avis, W.S., Drysdale, P.D., Gregg, R.J., Neufeldt, V.E., & Scargill, M.H. (1983). *Gage Canadian Dictionary*. Toronto, Canada: Gage Educational Publishing.

As a nursing or midwifery student entering the profession in the UK, you will be asked for a CV. In the US, the term used is résumé, and in Canada you will find both terms used. I have used CV here, but the advice is the same regardless of which you are asked for.

What goes into a CV?

There are very few rules about what sections must be on a CV. There is also no 'right' length. In general, you can expect your CV to be just 1–2 pages at the beginning of your career, and to expand as your work experience grows. The key requirements are:

- name and contact details;
- education (post-secondary only, unless you are in years 1–2 of a post-secondary program);
- professional licensing or certification;
- previous work (or volunteer) experience: you may wish to divide this into sections such as 'relevant experience' and 'additional experience';
- professional memberships, presentations;
- awards and honours;
- references.

You may also wish to include

- Objective[s]: if you are applying to a job that is specifically described in the ad, these are a good way of highlighting how your qualifications fit the requirements. If the nature of the job is not clear, however, you run the risk of defining yourself in a way that doesn't match what they are looking for. It might be better in that case just to let the CV speak for itself – if you get an interview, it is common at that time for interviewers to ask about your current career objectives and long-term goals.
- Skills: a list of skills can be impressive as a way to highlight specific or uncommon skills, if you know they are relevant to the job.

The following advice on CVs and job applications was written by Dr Margaret Procter, Coordinator of Writing Support at the University of Toronto. It has been slightly adapted to reflect nursing and midwifery situations.

Application letters and CVs: some practical tips

- **Keep the reader's interest in mind.** Your message is 'you need me', not 'I want a job'. Know enough about the organization or agency to recognize what they want and need. Then the focus of your documents will be where you fit and what you can contribute. This principle will also determine your choice of emphasis and even your wording (not 'I have had four months of clinical placement' but 'My clinical placement experience will help me do X and Y').
- **Balance facts and claims.** Your documents will be boring and meaningless if they're just bare lists of facts. They will be empty and unbelievable if they are just grand claims about yourself. Use each of the two or three paragraphs in the body of your letter to make a few key interpretive statements ('I enjoy working collaboratively with the community to meet their identified needs'). Back up each one with some examples. Were you responsible for any innovations, changes or improvements? They could be big (e.g., 'achieved community consensus to open a harms reduction injection site in a residential neighbourhood of MyCity') or small ('initiated new sharps disposal procedure on my unit').
- **Write concisely.** There is no space available for word-spinning. At the beginning of your career, you may feel your CV looks a little thin – don't try to pad it with unnecessary words and details.

Specific points about application letters

- Write a letter for each application, tailored for the specific situation. Even if the ad calls only for a CV, send a letter anyway. The letter makes a first impression, and it can direct the reader to notice key points of the CV.
- Use standard letter format, with internal addresses (spell names correctly!) and salutations. Use specific names or at least position titles whenever possible (call the organization or check its website). Most application letters for entry-level jobs are one page in length – a substantial page rather than a skimpy one.
- Start strong and clear. For an advertised position, name the job and any reference numbers, and say where you saw the ad. For a speculative letter, name a specific function you can perform and relate it to something you know about the organization.
- Use paragraph structure to lead your reader from one interpretive point to another. Refer to specific information in

terms of examples for the points you're making, and mention that your CV gives further evidence.

* End simply by thanking the reader for their consideration, and/or that you hope to have the opportunity to speak with them in an interview.

Specific points about CVs

* Have more than one on hand, emphasizing different aspects of your qualifications or aims. Then you can update and revise them quickly when opportunities arise.
* Make them easy to read by using headings, point form, and lots of white space. Look at current books of advice or at online templates to see the range of page formats available. Create one that suits your situation rather than following a standard one rigidly.
* The basic choice is between the traditional chronological organization (with the main sections Education and Experience) and the functional one (where sections name types of experience or qualities of character). You can get some of the benefits of both by creating a one- or two-line introductory section called *Profile* or *Objective* to sum up your main unifying point. You may also use *Achievement* subsections to emphasize your most important qualifications. These may include a horizontal list of keywords in noun form to serve in electronic scanning for information.
* List facts in reverse chronological order, with the most recent ones first. Shorten some lists by combining related entries (e.g., part-time jobs). In general, omit details of high-school achievements. You also don't have to include personal details or full information for referees.

Finally, here are some pitfalls to avoid:

* unsupported claims;
* large empty spaces (in this case, it's better to condense the CV);
* font sizes of less than 12 point;
* crowded pages (use white space between sections, and make headings clearly visible);
* errors in spelling and grammar;
* elaborate fonts or formatting.

Sources

Freedman, L. (2011). *Résumés FAQ*. Toronto, Canada: Health Sciences Writing Centre, University of Toronto.

Procter, M. (1999). *Application letters and résumés: Some practical tips*. Toronto, Canada: University of Toronto.

CLINICAL AND AGENCY DOCUMENTATION

Every practice setting has its own process and requirements for documentation, as well as its own 'shorthand' and accepted abbreviations for describing common phenomena. When you start a clinical or agency placement, be prepared to have a lengthy orientation to various unit or agency writing protocols; there will also be legal documents to sign.

You can expect to be trained both formally through training sessions and informally through colleagues, preceptors or mentors. The formal means of training you and evaluating your progress are explained during orientation. Getting informal training and feedback 'on the ground', however, is less straightforward than attending training sessions. That's because the quantity and quality are dependent on the culture of the particular practice setting.

By 'culture' we mean two things: first, it's the collective behaviour of the people who are part of an organization. This behaviour is shaped by the organization's values and goals, its working language, and its norms of practice. Second, culture is the behaviours and assumptions that are taught, formally and informally, to new members of the organization (Shein, 1992). A simple way to express it is, an organization's culture is 'the way things get done around here' (Deal & Kennedy, 2000).

For further reading

Deal, T. E., & Kennedy, A. A. (2000). *Corporate cultures: The rites and rituals of corporate life*. Harmondsworth: Perseus/Penguin.
Shein, E. (1992). *Organizational culture and leadership: A dynamic view*. San Francisco, CA: Jossey-Bass.

This means you may experience a highly supportive preceptorship/mentorship relationship, and professional colleagues who are willing and able to devote time to answering questions and helping out. Or, this may not be so. Either way, during orientation, you might ask who the best person is to ask for help with documentation, recording and other writing. Experience in the setting will also quickly show you which colleagues you can most comfortably ask for help.

The effectiveness of your clinical or agency writing is often determined by how other health professionals read and use it. What you document should facilitate clinical reasoning, and it should communicate your patient's clinical issues to all members of the health care team. In modern interprofessional and multidisciplinary practices, your care may intersect with any or all of the following on a regular basis: physicians of numerous specialties, social workers, educators, administrators, nutritionists and dietitians, occupational therapists, physical therapists, pharmacists, and others.

What is captured in clinical/agency documentation?

The specifics of what is captured are determined by the following factors:

- the nature and setting of the work being done;
- the purpose of the patient contact you are recording;

- the information you judge is relevant to include;
- the electronic health record (EHR) management system in use in your setting.

The timing of clinical/agency record-keeping

- Documentation is ideally done when the event occurs or as soon as possible thereafter. This is made easier in hospital settings with bedside terminals.
- PDA technology can be indispensable for nursing/midwifery work both within organizations and in community practice.
- Further documentation is done at end-of-shift for handover.

Recording professionally

- Write concisely: less really is 'more'.
- Write precisely: what do you really mean to say? Recording is not literature where the reading audience interprets meaning.
- Do not use shortened terms that are unlikely to be known. Have you seen or heard others in your practice setting use the acronyms and abbreviations?
- Keep in mind that there is a legal dimension to professional record-keeping. Failure to document properly can be the basis of legal action such as a lawsuit.

How recording is done

Recording methods vary across a spectrum from notes written in pen on a paper form to complex computerized charting systems that are highly integrated with other hospital functions. In these systems, data are entered via a combination of keyboarding and choice of touchscreen options. Integration of voice technology is not far off. You will be trained in whatever system your practice setting uses.

What gets recorded

Problem-oriented records are organized according to the patient's health problems. All health professionals involved in the patient's care contribute to and use the same record, allowing coordination of care from initial contact to discharge and follow-up at home. Two widely used formats (SOAP and PIE) are given below, but all problem-oriented approaches follow the same basic structure:

Data base	Contains initial health information.
Problem list	Consists of a numerical list of the patient's health problems.
Plan of care	Identifies methods for solving each health problem.
Progress notes	Describe the patient's responses to what has been done and revisions to the original plan (Timby, 2009, p. 112).

For further reading

Power, R. (2011, 14 Sept.). *Writing styles: Academic, professional and agency writing: The practice* [PowerPoint presentation]. University of Toronto: Factor-Inwentash Faculty of Social Work.

Timby, B. K. (2009). *Fundamental nursing skills and concepts* (9th ed.). Philadelphia: Wolters Kluwer Health/Lippincott Williams & Wilkins.

SOAP note format

The purpose of SOAP notes is to document a patient's presenting signs, symptoms and other information, to create a nursing diagnosis, and to provide a plan for treatment and care. SOAP notes provide a record to evaluate the success of treatment and care, and they form part of the patient's medical and legal record. In a lawsuit, SOAP notes can be introduced in court to provide a record of the health care team's diagnosis and treatment. To maintain the integrity of that record, corrections must be done in a way that does not obliterate the original.

Depending on the protocols of your setting, SOAP notes may be written in pen in the patient's medical record and/or entered in a computerized documentation system. They begin with a record of the initial information required within the practice setting. Usually, this is the individual's name, case number, today's date, and any procedure coding that may be required. Your organization is likely to have a manual on policy and procedure for clinical abbreviations.

As Shannon Abbaterusso, RN and clinical instructor, advises:

> There is usually a list of attached abbreviations that are approved by individual institutions and it is important that they are noted as they can differ quite significantly. Clinicians need to be careful about using abbreviations that they learn from other staff members as there are usually many that are frequently used and not approved. Esp., as we see in the downtown hospitals there are many physicians and agency nurses that move from hospital to hospital and may not be aware of the specific hospital's expectations. (personal communication)

Correct coding and abbreviations are crucial to preventing medication errors. This includes knowing when not to use them, so you will also receive standards for what *not* to use. For example, .1mg can be misread as 1mg, resulting in a 10-fold medication dosage error (you should write 0.1mg), while 10µg (micrograms) can be misread as 10mg (milligrams), leading to a 1000-fold dosage error (you should write 10mcg). In general, it is dangerous to use abbreviations for drug names because multiple drugs may have similar abbreviations.

1   Sentences are direct and short, and often incomplete.
2   Language is clear, precise, and descriptive. It uses technical terminology and approved abbreviations, but not jargon (i.e., any health professional on your team can understand it).

The body of the note is broken up into the following four sections:

S = Subjective: what the patient said

- the reason for the visit;
- symptoms being experienced: the location, onset, severity, duration, and frequency;
- history of presenting condition;
- past medical and social history;
- current medications;
- other notes, e.g., appetite, diet.

O = Objective: what you did and observed as a result

- Record measurements and vital signs, such as weight and height, blood pressure, pulse, oxygen saturation.
- Clinical examinations of the patient's body systems.
- Avoid opinion and record only the facts observed. Do not make subjective assumptions about the patient, for example, 'Mum appeared angry.' She may appear so to you but be feeling some quite different emotion.
- Do not make a diagnosis in this section: for example, 'Baby C exhibited all the signs and symptoms of MS' suggests you have decided on a diagnosis before you collect and analyze all your data.

A = Assessment or Analysis: evaluate the information you have obtained

- This section analyzes the subjective and objective notes and synthesizes them to create one or more nursing diagnoses.
- To make a diagnosis, identify what the patient is at 'risk for', 'related to' what, as 'evidenced by' what.
- List ongoing and new problems along with current status (stable, progressing, improved, resolved).

P = Plan:

- recommendations for further tests and assessments;
- relief measures or actions that worsen the patient's symptoms;
- recommendations for treatment (type, frequency, duration);
- medication changes (started, discontinued, increased, decreased);
- expected outcomes, short-term goals, long-term goals;
- referrals;
- recommendations for patient education and home instructions;
- discharge notes.

Many hospitals and agencies split **Plan** into more precise categories to create *soapie* or *soapier* notes:

Implementation: Care provided

Evaluation: Outcome of treatment

Revision: Changes in treatment

Note: there has been a strong movement in hospital settings towards computer charting. This form of charting is called **charting by exception.** As Timby (2009) describes it:

> Charting by exception is a documentation method in which nurses chart only abnormal assessment findings or care that deviates from the standard. Proponents of this efficient method say that charting by exception provides quick access to abnormal findings because it does not describe normal and routine information. (p. 114)

PIE notes (problem, intervention, evaluation) assign a number to each of a patient/ client's problems, and use the numbers subsequently as the notes progress through intervention and evaluation, for example, P#1, I#1, E#1, P#2, etc. There are a number of other variations, such as P-CARE (Patient, Clinician, Assessment, Results, Evaluation).

For further reading

Nursing and Midwifery Council. (2009). *Record-keeping: guidance for nurses and midwives.* London: NMC. Available at www.nmc-uk.org

Timby, B. K. (2009). *Fundamental nursing skills and concepts* (9th ed.). Philadelphia: Wolters Kluwer Health/Lippincott Williams & Wilkins.

WITNESS STATEMENTS

In the event of a lawsuit, a coroner's inquest, or for other reasons, nurses and midwives are sometimes required to make a statement or testify at a court hearing. It is important to be familiar with and understand the legal obligations and rights that are relevant to your jurisdiction. These can be found on the websites of your national and state/ provincial regulatory bodies. These bodies also stand ready to guide you in dealing with legal matters arising out of your professional practice.

The prospect of giving testimony in the unfamiliar and somewhat daunting environment of court is a challenge if you are not experienced in it. Luckily, lawyers are no more likely to let a new nurse or midwife stand unprepared before a hearing than you are to hand over your stethoscope and point a lawyer toward your patient's bed. If you have kept high-quality notes and records, they will not be difficult to organize into a witness statement. The contents of a witness statement are described here by Alexandra Mayeski, a lawyer who specializes in health law:

> Witness statements should summarize the evidence that is to be given at the hearing. The evidence should be first hand. They should provide

some background of the person and why that person is giving evidence. The evidence of the witness at the hearing will usually be limited to that which is in the statement so you want to make sure everything is covered. (personal communication)

WRITING FOR HEALTH EDUCATION

My favourite example of the seemingly unbridgeable gap between science and the public is a 10-year-old analysis of the difficulty of scientific language. In this study a standard English-language newspaper was given a rating of zero. Anything above zero was more difficult; anything below easier. The highest rating was 55.5, assigned to a paper in the journal *Nature*. In fact nothing scientific rated less than 28.

But adult fiction came in at –19.3 and adult-to-adult conversations (casual) were –41.1. The only categories ranked lower were mothers talking to their 3-year-olds (–48.3) and farmers talking to dairy cows (–59.1).

From Jay Ingram, 'Why science stories bomb with readers', *The Toronto Star*, Sunday, December 30, 2001, p. F8

'Health education' is a broad term that refers to the process of educating people about health. The goal is to give people the knowledge and skills they need to make quality health decisions, and to behave in a way that promotes, maintains, or restores their health. Health education can be directed toward individuals, groups, or communities. Considering the findings of the study Mr Ingram describes, it goes without saying that the language you use in writing for health education needs to be crystal clear. But according to whose definition of 'clear' are you writing? The answer depends on which community is your target.

'Community' may be defined geographically (e.g., the catchment area of a hospital or agency); ethnically (e.g., Hmung, San) or racially (e.g., African American); by residence (e.g., a housing development or a neighbourhood); by stage in life cycle (e.g., infants, teens, older adults); by common health concern (e.g., stroke, homelessness); by use of a particular health or social service resource (e.g., community clinic); by adherence to a particular health belief system (e.g., users of herbal medicines); adherence to a particular health behaviour (e.g., smokers, drinkers) or by some combination of these or other characteristics. It's important to take careful account of these and other intersecting factors in understanding the population you are writing for.

According to Bell (1995, p. 300), effective health education materials . . .

* remove obstacles to learning and make the learning process easier;
* are free of confusing language and irrelevant content;
* encourage feelings of competency and self-worth;
* respect and value the past experience of the reader;

- are designed to integrate new learning into the past experience of the reader;
- indicate an achievable, observable goal, along with practical actions and behaviours to achieve it;
- are tested and refined in collaboration with individuals or groups who represent the intended audience.

In health education materials, then, it is important to clearly identify and understand the community, or population, and either conduct a needs assessment or in some way ascertain the message you want to deliver. And then you will need to tailor the language and design elements you use so they are the most easily understood, most engaging, and most persuasive for that population.

It is often advised that health education materials be written with the use of a readability formula, such as the SMOG Readability Formula or the Gunning Fog Index. These various formulas – none of which were designed for the health professions – count the number of letters in words and words in sentences, or use other simple mathematical methods, and then produce a score intended to predict what grade level of education is needed to understand the written material. Unfortunately, such scoring reduces the multiple influences on the complex process of reading to the single dimension of grade level. It doesn't account for the fact that even while we are still in school, we all read at different levels. Or that in the multicultural societies of today's world, not all individuals have gone through the same school system or learned the same forms of English. It doesn't take account of the multiple life experiences outside school that may encourage us to read and learn, or act as a barrier to further learning. Finally, it ignores the fact that it is possible to be very confusing and dull while using short words and sentences.

This is not to say that readability formulas have no value. Bell (1995, p. 303) reminds us that there are a great many members of society who are low-skilled readers, and these formulas do focus writers of health education materials on the need to write simply. Another appeal of a focus on educational level is the fact that individuals with less education tend to have more health problems, and therefore to be very important targets for health education materials. However, readability formulas should be used with caution, as a guide to locate areas where you may wish to revise, not as a guide to the actual revision. That needs to be based on your analysis of the target audience, and on the input that you gather from them as part of the development process.

Beyond the reader's past experience, the other important determinant of the language you use is **context**, that is, the circumstances under which they are reading. For example, when surgical patients are discharged and given instruction sheets for self-care, the sheets inevitably contain medical language they might normally not be familiar with. But having gone through the illness and surgical experience, they are likely to understand the medical terminology around it (and part of good discharge planning, of course, is probing whether they are indeed understanding), as long as everything around the terminology – the sentence structures and word choices – is clear, simple and direct. Bear in mind that people often receive health education materials when they and their families are in crisis.

To achieve maximum readability for a general audience, consider the following questions.

What exactly am I asking people to do?

- Can I express it in a few, simple words?
- Why exactly should they do it? Have I explained this?
- What will happen if they don't? Have I explained this?

How likely are they to do it?

- What will empower them to act?
- Can they incorporate my suggestions into their day-to-day life?

What are the barriers they face?

- Do I offer easy, practical suggestions to overcome them?
- Do the changes I suggest fit in with my readers' lifestyle?

Have I chosen a small number of key words I want my readers to remember?

- Do I repeat one or more in every section?

Am I blaming people or empowering them?

- No one appreciates being nagged or lectured. For example, which of these would make you more likely to act?
  - o No one likes the fat kid in the class. As a parent, it is up to you to keep your child from obesity.
  - o As a parent, you can not control what your children eat at school. But here are a few simple ways to help them choose healthy foods.

What is my layout like?

- Is there plenty of white space between my visual 'blocks' of text and illustration? This helps set them out for the reader.
- Do my illustrations/visuals send the right message clearly?
- Do I use bulleted lists as well as paragraphs?
- Do I make key messages larger or set them out or place them first?

What kind of language am I using?

- Do I use short paragraphs (1-4 sentences)?
- Do I use short sentences (generally not more than 10-12 words)?
- Do I use common words and mostly short ones?

- Do I address the reader directly as 'you'? Compare the impact of these two:
  o Pain will be reduced within 24 hours.
  o You will feel less pain within a day.
- Do I use catchy phrases that are easy to remember? Consider, for example, which of these you yourself would find easier to remember?
  o You must seek treatment immediately or risk killing millions of brain cells.
  o Time equals brain cells.

COMMUNICATING ONLINE

Professional email communication and email etiquette

From: 8432x@server.com

To: busyprof@university.edu

Subject: Re:

Yo prof!

Did i miss anything thursday? Cn U pls send me yr notes! ☺

Joey

Clearly 'Joey' didn't attend Thursday's class. But was it the course Busyprof taught in the morning or was it the night class? Is Joey's full name Joseph or Josephine, JoAnn, Jonghua or even Jasmine? The email address is no help because the student hasn't used an institutional email account. An email account given you by your college or university will always include your name. Next, a professor who has just been disrespectfully addressed as 'Yo prof' isn't inclined to waste much time trying to figure any of this out. Finally, notice that Joey clearly believes it doesn't matter if she or he attends classes. Professors find it frustrating when students think that everything of value in a class is covered in PowerPoint slides and handouts.

Your aim in an email is to communicate clearly and efficiently, presenting a professional identity to the recipient. Here is a summary of the good, practical advice most commonly given about professional email communication:

- Some general points about emails:
  o One topic per email message – if you need to discuss two or more items, send two or more emails, with each topic identified in the subject line. Never leave the subject line blank, or write something meaningless like 'Hi.' If you are writing with a question about an assignment, say so: 'Question about MDW202 first assignment'.

- o   Keep your message short and to the point – unless you have a good reason for making it longer, your reader should be able to see the entire message on a single screen. This is to avoid a situation where a busy reader omits to scroll down and misses part of the message.
- o   Short paragraphs are easier to read than long ones.
- o   Be careful if you need to send sensitive information. Email is *not* a secure form of communication. If you need to include confidential or private information, make sure you encrypt the email. The simplest way to do this is to send the material in a password-protected attachment and to send the password in a separate email.
- o   Always proofread twice, slowly and carefully, before hitting 'send'.
- o   Never send an email when you are very upset about something to do with the recipient (e.g., a poor grade on a paper you worked hard on, or a colleague in your practice setting who failed to show up for a shift, making you work overtime). Wait at least a day. Write a draft if it makes you feel better, but keep your finger off that send button until you've revisited it and revised.
- Identify yourself properly:
  - o   Use your institutional email address, not a personal account. Personal accounts don't always include your name, but an institutional address will identify both your name and the organization where you study or work.
  - o   Always identify the key message of the email in the subject line, for example, 'Invitation to breastfeeding education session' or 'Questions re new intake process'.
  - o   Sign the message with your name and professional contact information. Don't add tag lines or quotes at the bottom. Don't include social media contacts such as a link to your Facebook account.
- Be courteous:
  - o   Unless you have a working relationship with the recipient, use formal modes of address (Prof., Dr., Mr., Ms, Sir/Madam). In North America, it is simply acceptable to use the person's full name (Dear JoAnn Kurtz).
  - o   Be patient if you don't receive an immediate reply – especially do not expect a fast reply to an email sent outside business hours.
- Respect confidentiality and privacy:
  - o   This cannot be overemphasized. In no area of your professional or personal life should you ever reveal identifying details of patients or clients.
  - o   Failure to respect confidentiality and privacy has both ethical and legal implications and may have serious consequences.

- Don't confuse social media with professional communication:
  - o Use full sentences, and check your spelling, grammar and punctuation.
  - o Don't type words or sentences in UPPERCASE – IT IS THE EQUIVALENT OF SHOUTING.
  - o Using all lowercase makes you seem lazy, as does omitting punctuation.
  - o Don't use emoticons such as smiley faces.
  - o Don't use abbreviations such as 'lol' or 'u' for 'you'.
  - o Don't include unsolicited, non-professional attachments, such as trip photos or YouTube videos.
- Replying to emails:
  - o Reply promptly, ideally the same day, even if it's only to acknowledge receipt and say that you will respond more fully later. However, if you receive a professional communication outside business hours or on the weekend, do not feel obliged to reply until regular working hours.
  - o Include the original message so the recipient has the context for your reply.
  - o If you have been asked a number of questions, make sure you clearly identify and answer them all.
  - o If others were copied on the original, make sure you are comfortable with everyone on the list reading your reply. If not, check and double-check to make sure your cursor is poised over 'reply' and not 'reply-all'.

Discussion boards, chatrooms, blogs, and other online forums

Increasingly, nursing programs are adapting social media for use within the course context, even assigning marks for (meaningful) participation in online forums. Learning to use social media is also excellent training if your goal is community practice as a nurse or midwife, when you may want to use email and social media to communicate with clients, or use websites for health promotion purposes. Currently, the most common online forums used in courses are discussion boards, chatrooms, and blogs.

Some cautions: within the course context, social media cease to be only a form of personal expression and assume a greater degree of formality. Be careful not to include opinions and details that you wouldn't mention in a face-to-face tutorial group. These include details about patients or healthcare settings that could identify them; sensitive or confidential information; negative 'venting' about instructors, courses or practice settings or preceptors.

An excellent source of guidance on using social media for nursing and midwifery is:

Fraser, R. (2011). *The nurse's social media advantage: How making connections and sharing ideas can enhance your nursing practice*. Indianapolis, IN: Sigma Theta Tau International Honor Society of Nursing.

SUCCESSFUL PRESENTATIONS 10

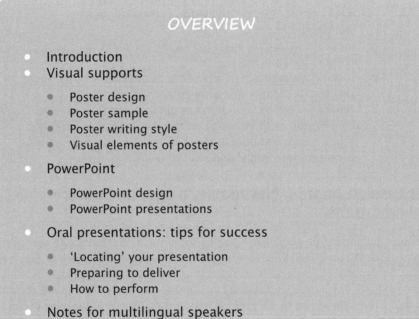

In this chapter, we will consider:

- writing, design, and oral communication skills for successful presentations;
- what to include and how to organize it;
- how to support presentations with well-designed posters or PowerPoint;

- the strategies used by engaging, informative presenters;
- some special challenges facing multilingual presenters;
- some special challenges of group presentations.

INTRODUCTION

You may be asked to make a presentation to your class on a course-related topic, or to your colleagues in your practice setting or agency, or as part of a research day. These presentations often include some interactive element such as a discussion or activity or audience questions. The visual supports you use may be paper-based, such as a flip chart, posterboard, overhead transparencies, or printed handouts. Or they may be computer-based (such as PowerPoint or online handouts). There will a set length of time for speaking, which can range from five minutes up to an hour. You may be asked to present individually or as part of a group. You can generally expect that the audience will ask you questions at the end.

Presentations always contain a verbal element and a visual element, but the proportions vary. For example, a PowerPoint presentation is a talk supported by slides. A poster is a visual presentation supported by a short explanatory talk, often to a panel of judges.

A presentation is a summary of the most important information you decide your audience needs to know about some larger topic. The content and organization vary according to the topic and your purpose in presenting it. For example, the purpose of the sample poster in Figure 10.1 is to report the results of a nursing student's literature review on needle exchange programmes and HIV, and it was done as a course assignment. As a result, the poster includes a lot of text organized into short paragraphs in fairly uniform columns. Because a presentation is a summary, you always know much more about the topic than you can include. This means making careful choices about what to include or leave out based on how much time you have and what your audience needs to be told.

Like any other piece of writing, a presentation has an introduction, a body, and a conclusion. But it doesn't get written in the same iterative way described in Chapter 3; instead, it is written as an outline of points, major and supporting, that are then fleshed out with evidence and comment as needed.

VISUAL SUPPORTS

Visual supports help you to reinforce key points in your presentation and provide supporting evidence and illustrations. The most traditional and simplest visual supports are chalkboards, dry-erase boards, and flip-chart pads, all of which you write or draw on as you present. We don't cover them here, as there is little to say beyond making sure your writing is large, clear, and dark enough to be seen from anywhere in the room.

Posters are commonly asked for as presentations at research days or poster conferences. PowerPoint presentation software allows you to prepare a multi-media slide display that can include text slides, sound and video clips, illustrations and photos. A more traditional form of slide presentation uses overhead transparencies and a projector. Transparencies are not as versatile as PowerPoint but have the advantage that you can write on them as you talk. But we begin with posters, which are commonly used in presentations before a small audience or displayed as part of a research day.

Poster design

Size: There are no rules for the exact size of a poster, but if you are given specific guidelines for dimensions, make sure you follow them carefully.

Materials: Poster boards are available in standard sizes at office supply stores. Software is available that allows you to design and print your poster as a single sheet, or you can use your computer's standard word processor to produce a series of letter-sized sheets (8 1/2" x 11" or A4) and affix them as panels to the poster board.

Layout: There are no rules for exact layout of a poster, but you should choose an overall layout that suggests an arrangement of communication areas. Some common options are:

- Top-to-bottom, left-to-right flow of information in vertical columns.
- Two fields in contrast.
- A centred set of images or data (tables and figures) flanked with columns of text.
- A centred set of images, data or text circled by text or visual blocks.
- Leave sufficient white space to create distinct communication areas. Test this by standing back from your poster far enough that you can't read the text – do the white areas clearly define blocks of text and image?
- Label figures and tables clearly and descriptively.
- Use large typeface. The following point sizes are recommended:

Title: 96

Subtitle: 24 point to 36 point

18 point for text

Don't use more than two fonts throughout. Also, don't mix serif and sans serif fonts (serif fonts have the little lines on the ends of the strokes that make up the letters; sans serif fonts don't):

Times New Roman   Arial

Be creative, but don't overdo the formatting to the extent that it obscures the information.

DO NOT WRITE ALL IN CAPITALS. IT IS IRRITATING.

Poster Sample

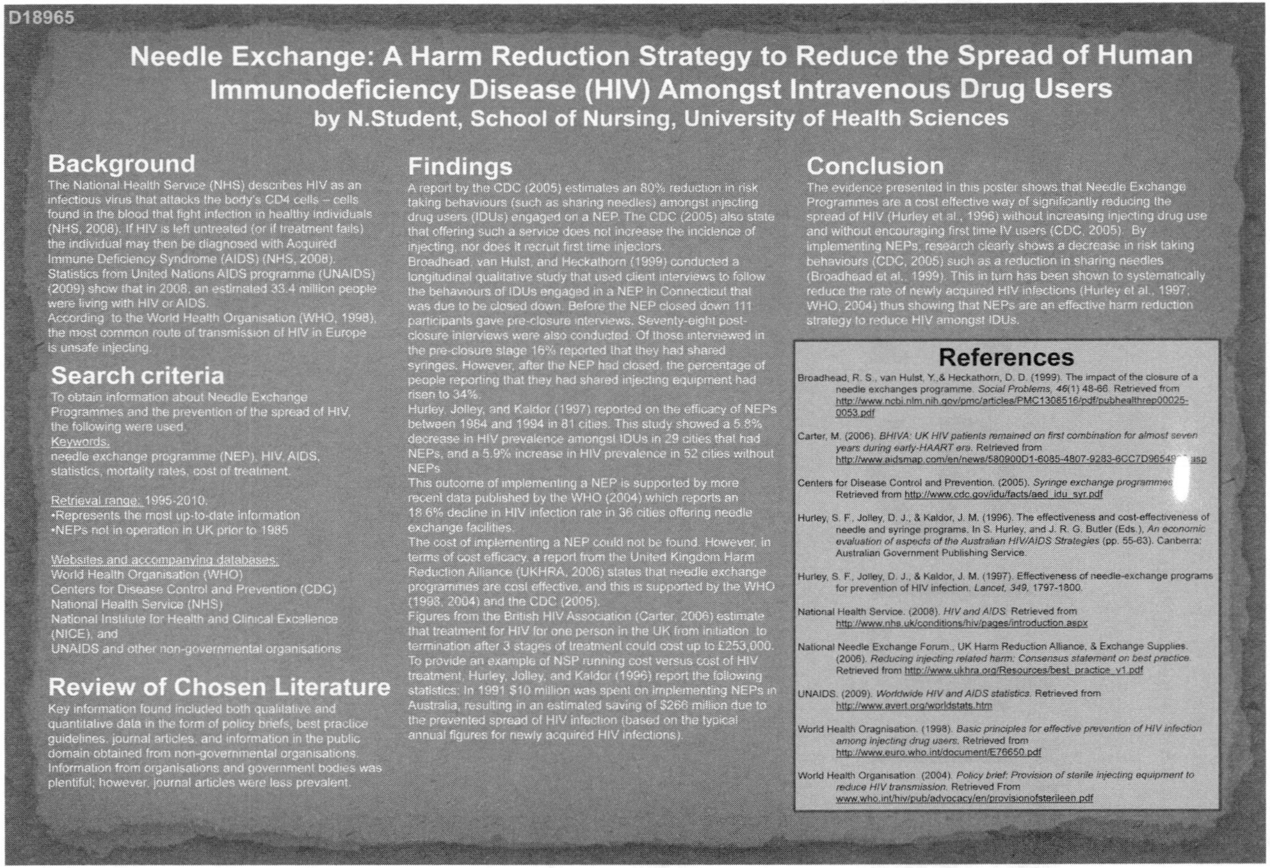

Figure 10.1 Poster on an evidence-based nursing intervention

Poster writing style

You need to maximize the limited space on a poster by writing in a style that is dense with information. This section will show you some ways to minimize the number of linking words in your sentences in favour of substance words. Keep in mind, though, that your writing also needs to be crystal clear to the reader, and balancing density with clarity isn't always easy.

A poster has to be self-contained:

- define all acronyms and abbreviations (except standard units of measurement);
- define unique or unusual terms the first time you use them.

Save space wherever possible: use digits for numbers unless the number begins a sentence. Abbreviate whenever possible, such as 'vs.' for 'versus' or 'e.g.' instead of 'for example'.

You can also compress your sentences by using lists and 'gapping', a technique in which all non-essential words are removed. Compression is especially useful in sections that give information. For example, the 'Search Criteria' section of Poster Sample A could be compressed this way:

Search criteria

Key words used: needle exchange programme (NEP), HIV, AIDS, statistics, mortality rates, cost of treatment.

Sources searched: WHO, Centre for Disease (CDC), National Institute for Health and Clinical Excellence (NICE), charitable organization websites (e.g., UNAIDS).

Dates searched: 1995–2010.

- Why this range?
  - NEPs not in operation in the UK until 1985.
  - 1995–2010 represents the most up-to-date information.

Visual elements of posters

The visual elements on a poster can include tables, figures (defined below), and any formatting elements that help to highlight the different sections of the poster. In general, try to keep the formatting elements as simple as possible. Too much detail and variety confuses and distracts the viewer from getting the message about what is most important.

As with text, where we signal importance through position and length, we have a number of ways to signal the relative importance of visual elements. Viewers expect information in the foreground to be more important than information in the background or on the periphery. They expect large visuals to be more important than small ones. They also expect things with the same size, shape, location or colour to be related to each other. Take advantage of this in designing your own layout.

Tables: Tables are used to display a body of related data so we can easily see changes and make comparisons. Make sure you refer to your tables within the text and explain why you are including them. The title of the table (always located *above* the table) needs to be clearly descriptive of the message of the table.

Figures: Anything that isn't a table is classified as a figure. Here are some of the most common types and what we use them for:

Photograph or drawing	To show what something looks like
Map	To show where something is located
Diagram	To show how something is put together
Line graph	To show the relationships between two or more sets of data plotted on a grid created by horizontal and vertical axes
Bar graph	Like a line graph, these plot a series of values on two axes, but using bars instead of points joined by a line. Each bar represents a quantity of something. Used to compare quantities and show trends
Flow chart	To show the sequence of steps in a process
Organizational chart	To show the vertical and horizontal structures of an organization
Pie chart	To show proportions and percentages

As with a table, you must refer to your figure within the text and explain why you are including it. Also, make sure that the caption (always located *below* the figure) describes the message of the figure very clearly.

POWERPOINT

PowerPoint design

PowerPoint software and others like it allow you to create digital slides which you project through an LCD projector and control through a computer. The basic structure is as follows:

Title slide: title of your presentation, your name and affiliation

Overview slide: point form outline of what you will be presenting

Introductory slides:

- background on your topic;
- why the topic is important;
- previous approaches;
- your approach.

Body

Concluding slides:

- clear statement of the overall message of your presentation;
- a look ahead [optional];
- acknowledgments [optional];
- consider designing an interesting final slide that can remain on-screen while you take questions, such as a photo representing your topic.

PowerPoint slides should be visually interesting but not overwhelming:

- Use bulleted points and parallel constructions [test 1...test 2... test 3].
- Use an Arial font, at least 16 point, **bolded.**
- For tables and figures, make sure the reproduction is clear and large enough to read. It is easiest to read tables in black text on a very light background. Include only one complex or two simple tables/figures per slide.
- Don't overcrowd but do fill the frame – no tiny objects in the middle of an empty screen.
- Don't overdo multiple colours and whizzing objects.
- Viewers with colour blindness will be disadvantaged if you use two colours based on the same primary colour (e.g., pink lettering on a red background, orange on yellow, or green on blue).

PowerPoint presentations

Some wag once noted that the big advance of PowerPoint is that it lets the audience sleep in the dark. Don't let that be your presentation!

Keep the introduction short. Tell your audience clearly and concisely what you are going to cover, and then get right into things while they (and you) are at their freshest. 'Taking command' in this way also helps you psychologically to get past any nervousness you've been feeling.

Focus on the critical points. You can amplify during the question period.

Use wording that establishes a hierarchy of importance, as well as numerical listings: 'The most important factor in the recent rise in TB cases has been … Two other factors that have had an impact are, first, … and second …'.

As you come to specialized terminology, define any terms you believe will not be known to your audience.

Announce your graphics, and if the content of the slides is not self-explanatory, explain it. Don't be the presenter who flips through slides without a word of explanation, sublime in the misconception that what is crystal clear to her or himself will be equally clear to the audience. On the other hand, don't be the presenter who laboriously reads every word of text on the slides and elaborates on each number and image. Instead, train yourself to engage with your slides when necessary but not otherwise: in your speaking notes, highlight the points at which you will turn briefly to the slide and gesture, using words (*not* a laser pointer) to direct the viewers' attention. Indicate both location (e.g., 'the table on the right gives values for...') and meaning (e.g., 'in this video clip we see a typical client interaction').

Always end at the end. That is, if you're running out of time, skip to the end. If you've rehearsed properly, this shouldn't happen but sometimes the unexpected surprises us – problems with equipment, for example, or a program day that is running behind time.

ORAL PRESENTATIONS: TIPS FOR SUCCESS

Some presenters write a paper and read their presentation verbatim from the prepared text (or even recite it from memory). I attended one session where the presenter also handed round copies of the text so we could read along – it was the longest 30 minutes of my life. Presenters use these strategies because they fear they will freeze up in front of an audience. They worry about being asked a question and not knowing – or not remembering – the answer. But unless you are a very fine actor, you will find it surprisingly difficult to deliver a prepared text with the fluidity of natural speech and you risk quickly losing the interest of your audience.

A better strategy is to write up a detailed outline that includes both paragraphs and bullet points and to train yourself – through as much rehearsal as you can possibly squeeze in – to speak from that instead of a fully prepared text. It isn't difficult to build a presentation outline:

- Use one side of the page only and number every page clearly. Leave a great deal of white space.
- Make headings larger and bolder.
- Lay out your points and supporting evidence using a combination of short paragraphs and multilevel bulleted points.
- Underline key words or ideas you will want to emphasize.
- As you practise speaking from your outline, mark cues on the text for pauses. Pauses create emphasis. They also help you remember to breathe!
- Mark cues for referring to your slides.

Use these principles to guide you in structuring speaking notes and deciding what to include:

1 The introduction should (if necessary) introduce yourself. Then say why you are making this presentation (e.g., to report on an existing program or intervention; to argue for a new program or intervention); outline what the presentation will cover; and give any background or definitions the audience will need.

2   The body of your talk should be clearly divided into sections that each present a single major point with arguments and/or visuals to support it. The amount of space and time given to individual sections should reflect their importance in relation to your overall purpose and topic. If your purpose is to present a review of the literature on the topic of pain management interventions for neonates, your largest section will be devoted to a summary and evaluation of the research literature, subdivided into the different categories or strengths of research evidence. Is your purpose to propose a new agency in a priority neighbourhood? – you will want to give the most space to identifying the issues in the neighbourhood and how this particular initiative will address them.

3   The conclusion should summarize the content and main argument of the presentation. The final section usually gives recommendations for research, theory, and/or practice. If relevant, end with a brief list of acknowledgments (two or three individuals or organizations that assisted you with information, funding, or technical/research support).

The audience at a presentation is not a passive entity. The individuals who make it up will be responding to your performance and it will show in their faces and body language. You can train yourself to make use of this. Many presenters find it helpful, as they come up to face the audience and begin to speak, to focus on the friendly, interested faces – especially their friends. As time goes on, it will be easier to observe the audience as you speak and make occasional eye contact. As you proceed, you will feel an overall sense emanating from the room: interest and enjoyment, or perhaps boredom and confusion.

The audience will also engage actively with you through questions and discussion. Generally this happens at the end of your presentation. In some presentation settings, such as a class, you may be able to pause at points to ask if anyone has questions or comments. If you are in a large room or auditorium, when someone asks a question, repeat it loudly and clearly – many in the audience will not have heard it. Doing so also gives your brain time to organize your answer.

Think of presenting as a type of theatre. You are there not just to inform but to do so in a way that engages – even entertains – your audience.

'Locating' your presentation

*   What is the physical space like in terms of size, shape, seating, lighting? Where are you standing within that space? Imagine how different it would be to present in these two common presentation settings:

    o   A classroom or seminar room with seating for 20–25 around a long, rectangular table. You stand at the head of the table and don't need a microphone. There is some light in the room even when darkened for PowerPoint, which is projected onto a small screen on the wall.

Or you may present using a poster and/or flip chart, which everyone can see easily. You can make eye contact easily and observe the audience's reactions to what you say. You can also move around the room if you need to.

o   An auditorium with seating for 100–200. The presentation area is at the bottom of a pit and the seating is raked (i.e., rows of seats rise at an angle so much of audience looks down at you). The presentation area is lit; the rest of the auditorium is darkened so you cannot see anyone clearly. You stand behind a fixed lectern in a corner beside the screen and speak into a microphone attached to the lectern. Your presentation is projected onto a large screen behind you.

* What are the acoustics like in the room? Acoustical quality is determined by a number of factors: the shape and dimensions of the room, the height of the ceiling, the materials used to build the room, the number and arrangement of people and furniture, and where you stand within the room.

* How good is the lighting? Are you in a room with windows letting in natural light that must be blocked so a screen can be used for PowerPoint? Is it an inner room with artificial lighting? Is the room uniformly lit or can portions of it be darkened (which allows slides to be seen while the audience has light to make notes by)? Or is the presentation area lit while the audience is in darkness, as in a theatre?

* What equipment is available to you and how good is the quality? Is technical support available in case of equipment problems?

* If you will be using a microphone, what kind is it? Is it fixed to a podium or lectern (you have no mobility); is it a 'stem' microphone that cradles on top of a stand and can be removed and held in your hand (you can choose whether to stand still or move around, but you lose use of one hand to do so)? Is it a microphone that you clip onto your clothing with a battery pack that clips onto your belt or waistband (you have complete mobility)? Or is the whole presentation area wired for sound (complete mobility)?

When you are using a microphone, speak at your normal volume. If you hear popping or a screeching noise, lower your voice or stand back a little. If you are not using a microphone, pause a few seconds into your presentation to ask those at the back of the room if they can hear you.

* Where will you be standing in the room? Will you be behind a lectern or free to move around? The ideal position is where the audience can see you and the screen at the same time, you don't block anyone's view, and you can easily operate a projector or computer.

- Is it a space you are well acquainted with (such as your usual classroom)? If not, can you go in ahead of time to familiarize yourself?

Preparing to deliver

You cannot rehearse too much or too often, and you should practise with a focus on developing three areas: clear, fluid delivery of your talk; a comfortable stage presence; and facility with using the technology of your visual supports.

- Rehearse, rehearse, rehearse. Spend extra time on the introduction, as this is the part where nervousness is most likely to make you stumble.
- Time yourself.
- Try to rehearse in a setting that approximates where you will be presenting or, if you can't, imagine yourself in such a space. Stand in the position you will occupy in the room.
- Ask a colleague, friend or family member to watch you rehearse. Ask them if you have any nervous gestures or recurring speech patterns that distract them from what you are saying, or are even annoying. Do you sway from side to side or back and forth? Do you fidget with your clothing or jewellery? Ask them to ask you questions at the end – every person who rehearses with you will have some different questions and some that will be the same, which will give you some idea of what you are most likely to be asked. The questions they ask will sometimes surprise you, things you hadn't thought of – and now you're prepared for them.
- Make sure you learn how to operate any technology you'll be using and rehearse with it until it becomes a seamless part of your talk.
- Make up a list of questions you might be asked. Imagine an audience in front of you. Imagine them asking you the questions. Answer out loud as if they were there.
- Practise safe redundancy – bring backup copies of your presentation using a different technology. For example, you can bring a PowerPoint presentation on both a notebook computer and a USB key. You can also email it to yourself ahead of time and retrieve the presentation directly into an on-site system in case your own computer fails to connect with the system.
- Bring whatever physical aids you might need, for example, throat lozenges, tissues, and a recyclable bottle of water.
- Get plenty of sleep.
- Avoid caffeine, but do hydrate with water.
- Dress professionally. Understand that your audience is not just judging your presentation – they are looking to see what kind of professional you are becoming. But also dress comfortably – now is not the time for new shoes. Even if they are comfortable, their newness is a distraction.

- Hold nothing in your hands except your notes. Especially avoid laser pointers – nothing conveys nervous energy more than a twitchy red dot jiggling across the screen. Use hand gestures and language instead: 'The mortality rates in the middle column of this table ...'.
- Don't bury your hands in your pockets or clutch a lectern – use them to gesture.

Don't worry if you feel nervous. That just makes you more nervous. It is natural to experience stage fright and many experienced presenters still feel twinges before they 'go on'. In the vast majority of cases the things we fear – freezing up, making some disastrous error, the audience hating our talk, etc. – never happen and the nervousness itself fades very quickly once we start. As well, the more rehearsing you have done, the more secure you will feel. It also helps to make a conscious effort to breathe and relax. Relaxation is cumulative – as you learn to do it, it gets easier until it becomes a habit. Here are a couple of relaxation exercises to get you started:

- Drop your hands to your sides; let them hang inert, dead weight; let them feel so heavy you don't think you can lift them. Do this anytime you can, such as on transit, or relaxing at night. When you've gotten good at relaxing your hands, move on to learning to relax your shoulders and neck. Shoulders and neck tend to be the spots where nervous tension collects first.
- Practise breathing, something you can do anywhere at any time. Become deeply aware of the fact that you are breathing – feel your lungs rise and fall as if a tide is coming in and out. Relax your throat and feel the air rushing through. Open your mouth and throat wide as if in a yawn (it's even better if you can make yourself yawn). Keep that openness and relaxed feeling as you exhale. Be so open and relaxed that air can come through both mouth and nose at the same time. Track the air down to the base of your lungs – feel your belly fill out and your ribs strain against your back muscles.

How to perform

These tips are based on the voice training that singers and actors receive to help them achieve a comfortable stage presence and a clear, strong delivery. Mental exercises reduce nervousness and increase confidence. Physical exercises provide stamina and increase the volume and clarity of your voice.

- Here is an exercise to relax you for the start of your talk. It will also oxygenate you and strengthen your speaking voice: In the minute before you go on, become aware of your breathing, in and out slowly, as deeply as is comfortable. Once you are standing in position, take a few seconds for a last comfortable breath, let it out, and take a normal intake. Hold your head high and look around the room as you begin to speak.

- Some people feel 'safer' if they stand close to a fixed object such as a lectern or console, perhaps touching the object occasionally to help with the sense of being grounded. Other people are more comfortable if they can move about the presentation area and gesture freely (but not excessively) with their arms and hands. In this way, we all have our own comfort levels, as long as we avoid the extremes of rigidity and wild movement.
- Begin S-L-O-W-L-Y: You will naturally speed up as you speak, especially if you are nervous. The slowness may sound awkward to you, but to the audience you will seem deliberate and confident.
- Speak to the whole room. Make eye contact.
- Project your voice to the back of the room or auditorium: in other words, lift your chin so that your throat is extended but not uncomfortably so. Look to the back of the room and, as you speak, imagine waves of sound travelling in a high arc right to the back row of seats. This psychological exercise will have a physiological effect, helping your voice to travel for a longer distance.
- Don't swallow your consonants: North Americans especially can be guilty of lengthening their vowels and sliding over consonants, often running words together or dropping final consonants altogether. The overall effect is that the audience can miss important words, or need to strain to understand what you are saying. A good exercise in rehearsal is to overemphasize final consonants to the point that they sound overly noticeable to you. If you listen carefully to actors on television or movies, you will notice that they 'overpronounce' their final consonants in this way.
- Don't let your good habits fall away as you near the end of your talk – before starting your conclusion, pause, take a comfortable breath, and articulate clearly as you signal the coming end. Use phrases such as 'In summary,...' or 'To conclude with some recommendations,...'.
- Body movements can work either for or against you. Fidgeting nervously with jewellery or tugging on clothing will distract your audience from your presentation. On the other hand, gesturing with your hands at the same time as you emphasize key words creates interest and facilitates understanding. Turning your head so you end up looking at every section of the audience instead of facing rigidly ahead allows you to face every member of your audience and include them all. Do this even if the lighting in the room is directed toward you so that you can't actually see the audience. After all, the audience doesn't know you can't see them.

NOTES FOR MULTILINGUAL SPEAKERS

Many students whose first language is not English, and who have not yet learned to be proficient in the language, lack confidence in their ability to lead a discussion and respond to questions. They worry about not understanding what others say or ask, or they worry that others won't understand them accurately. They find it challenging to understand the idiomatic speech of the native speakers in their courses, or the array of global accents among their colleagues in today's multicultural classes.

Many English language learners worry that, under time pressure to respond to questions, they won't find the words to express their ideas clearly and are concerned about making grammar mistakes. Or they worry because they need time to think of answers in their first language and mentally translate into English. (One of the strategies of successful English learners is to spend a few minutes each night thinking *in English* about what happened to them that day, or repeating out loud *in English* things they have learned or read.)

A few tips:

- Don't be afraid to ask people to clarify what they've asked (e.g., 'I'm not sure I caught your meaning'), especially if they've used some idiomatic expression or made some cultural reference you don't know. You will find people are generally happy to explain.
- Don't feel you need to answer quickly. Take a few seconds to think through your response. The audience isn't going anywhere; they will wait.
- Don't feel you need to speak quickly. Slow speech sounds deliberate and thoughtful, and also allows the audience time to absorb what you are saying.

GROUP PRESENTATIONS

This chapter has consistently spoken as though you are presenting alone, but you may be asked to make a collaborative presentation in which you present as a member of a group. Group presentations differ because they add a social dimension.

Your goal is to maximize the contributions of each participant while minimizing the possibility of interpersonal conflicts. A clear planning process will smooth your path.

In your first meeting, explore how much knowledge and what kind of knowledge each person brings to the group (e.g., one individual is a very strong writer/editor; another has clinical experience with the topic; a third works well with multimedia). At the same meeting, decide on a timeline and schedule of meetings. Also, decide on specific roles for each member, such as editor or facilitator (the person who coordinates what individual members are doing and checks on their progress). One individual should record all this and circulate it afterward to the group, so there is no confusion (or contention) later on about when and what everyone is to do.

A frequent question is whether it is better for each person to work independently on separate sections and to send their material, after an agreed-on period of time, to the selected editor of the group for melding into a single piece. We could call this the 'All-to-one' method (Collins & Bosley, 1995). Often the poor editor must then go chasing the inevitable one (or more!) who fails to send the work on time, or who has done a bad job, or done the wrong job. Another problem is that pieces written separately by individuals with different writing styles don't always meld easily. The editor may end up having to do a major rewrite, which may not sit well with the original writer and adds unfairly to the editor's workload.

Another editing pattern is the 'All-to-All' strategy, where the group works collaboratively from start to finish, sitting together for lengthy research, writing and editing sessions. Composition by committee, as it were. Unfortunately, interpersonal conflicts can quickly arise. Writing by committee is also time-intensive and hard to schedule.

So, to sum up the problems, collaborative work is time-consuming, hard to schedule, and can lead to conflict. On the other hand, leaving everyone on their own for too long can result in widely disparate pieces that don't connect in topic or style.

Two other editing patterns identified by Collins and Bosley (1995) are worth considering instead: the 'One-to-One-to-One' pattern, in which one member drafts a part and passes it to a second, who edits and passes it to a third, etc. Everyone edits, but the final person should be the 'senior editor' who can evaluate and incorporate the best feedback and put all the sections together. Finally, there is the 'All-to-One-to-One' pattern, where everyone writes individual parts and the editing is split between a content editor and a grammar/style editor.

When it comes to preparing for the oral presentation, each member should practise on her or his own, but it is wise to schedule at least two group rehearsals. Rehearse using your visuals, ideally in the space where you will be presenting. If you are all going to take part in the presentations, set firm time limits for each person and enforce them during group rehearsals. One of the best lessons I ever learned was from one professor who came to our first presentation class equipped with an egg timer. He overturned it at the start of the first student's presentation, and cut the student off with a curt 'Thank you, that will be all' the instant the sand finished running through. At the second presentation class, we were all finishing on time.

It is important to establish a harmonious atmosphere when you are working in a group. Given the stresses each member experiences balancing school and personal demands, tempers can flare and small disagreements can be become turf wars and personal disputes. Be polite, listen respectfully and carefully to the other participants' ideas. Try to seek agreement rather than dwell on differences of opinion. Be willing to compromise – a group working together can produce more and better results than the sum of the work individuals would produce.

For further reading

Collins, C. E., & Bosley, D. S. (1995). *Technical communication at work*. FortWorth, TX: Harcourt Brace College.

Quitman Troyka, L., & Hesse, D. (2007). *Simon & Schuster quick access reference for writers* (3rd Canadian ed.). Toronto: Pearson/Prentice Hall.

REFLECTIVE WRITING 11

WRITING AND THE REFLECTIVE PRACTITIONER

One of the dictionary definitions of the word 'reflect' is 'to think carefully'. Another, interestingly, is 'to bend back or fold back', such as light. When we engage in personal reflection, we shine a light into ourselves, into our own experiences and actions, as well as into our own position within our professions and our society as a whole.

In the same way that caring for one's self is an essential component of caring for others, understanding ourselves is essential for understanding others. Self-reflection develops self-awareness, through which we learn to place value on the lives and experiences (what we call the 'lived experience') of others. That understanding creates the empathy and human connection which allow us to care for our patients.

Humans are creatures who 'self-interpret', that is, we are always in the process of creating meaning out of the situations we find ourselves in. As we become aware of what constitutes our own personal and social worlds, we become sensitive to the clues (words, actions, emotions) by which our patients and their families define their own worlds and their health.

For the reflective practitioner, events and how we act within them lead to reflection. Reflection leads to awareness, prompting further decisions on action or changes in practice.

What is reflective writing?

Reflective writing asks you to capture on paper your thoughts, your reflections, about the new events you experience in your practice and the new knowledge you are exposed to in your academic studies. It also forces you to focus on developing an awareness of who *you* are as you begin your program and how you change as you move through it.

Reflective writing assignments fall on a spectrum that ranges from:

- The highly personal, where you reflect on an event you experienced in your practice, with no reference to course readings or lectures, to . . .
- A mid-ground, where you reflect on personal experience in the context of the readings and lectures, as well as the larger objectives of the course. And finally, . . .
- The highly academic, where you are discussing the course readings with only minimal relation to personal experience.

When you start an assignment, ask yourself where on this spectrum it fits. Then organize your paper accordingly to provide more or less focus on the personal and academic elements.

You will also encounter some of the authors in your course readings engaging in reflective writing. Reflective writing has an important role within the qualitative stream of research. As we saw in Chapter 8, when you read qualitative studies, you will frequently find sections in which the researchers 'locate' themselves socioculturally and reflect on their relationship to their subject matter and the individuals whose lives they explore to answer their research questions.

You can also make important use of reflection in your practice, by encouraging your patients to engage in self-reflection. An exciting way to help patients through reflection is by means of art. Increasingly, both hospital and long-term care settings are creating special displays of the writing and artwork of patients. Through writing stories and poems, or through drawings and photos, or through posters which incorporate multiple forms of creative expression, your patients can express who they are, what they are experiencing, what their hopes are, who and what matters to them in life. In this way, they strengthen their own sense of personal identity, which becomes compromised when people enter health care institutions. Further, they become known – as individuals instead of only as medical cases – to the health providers who are part of their lives for days, months, or years.

The benefits of reflective writing

- Reflective writing engages you in a different type of learning from what you engage in when you memorize facts or statistics in order to give them back to the professor on exams. The learning that occurs through reflective writing is deep, personalized, and long-lasting.

- It opens a dialogue with course and clinical instructors through their responses to your writing.
- Reflection helps you move beyond *received knowledge* (what does the lecturer say? What do the readings say? What does the marker want to see in my papers and tests?) to *constructed knowledge* (how do *I* relate what I'm learning to my experience? What can *I* bring to my practice and my profession?).
- It helps you think about the way you are as a person rather than just what you do for a job.
- It helps you develop *conceptual* thinking (e.g., how does poverty affect the ability to cope with illness?) instead of only *fact-based* thinking (e.g., the most effective hand-washing technique).
- It helps you get past 'right' and 'wrong' in communicating your ideas about human behaviour and interactions.
- It helps foster caring (i.e., the ability to understand and express the perspective and concerns of your patients and their lived experience; to expand your own perspective).
- It helps develop a wider world-view. It forces you to challenge views and ideas you (and society) have accepted without question. Reflection is a personal journey, and it is not always an easy one. You may realize some things about yourself, the health care system, or the society you live in that you don't like.
- It promotes an understanding of diversity in culture, values, and behaviour.
- It raises questions, though it doesn't always provide answers.

A note on personal pronouns in reflective writing

Your professors recognize that students bring many valuable life experiences and skills with them into a course of study. They want to help you learn to have the confidence to apply that rich experience to your professional life.

At the same time as you use your writing to develop an authentic personal style, though, that writing is being done within the rigours of academic work. Writing assignments will usually ask you to 'integrate' research and/or theory with your experience. The goal is to combine the two in a way that adds to our understanding of both. How, though, do you do this?

1   You **don't** do it by expressing a simple personal opinion about the research. You wouldn't, for example, say something like:

Mishel and Braden are right when they describe their theory of uncertainty.

2   You **don't** do it just by putting your experience side-by-side with a statement about the research:

> The patient demonstrated Mishel and Braden's theory of uncertainty when she grew very fearful. This theory states that '[a long quoted sentence from Mishel & Braden]'.

This doesn't work because there isn't any real connection between the two. What is it about 'very fearful' that suggests uncertainty? Also, how does the writer know the patient was fearful?

What, then, does an authentic personal style look like?

1   It uses personal pronouns (I, me, my) to describe the personal experience, your reactions to it, how you would change your practice in future. It is possible that you may be asked *not* to use personal pronouns in reflective writing assignments, but that is unusual. It makes for very awkward writing when you have to refer to yourself indirectly while telling the story of events you have been part of. So, unless you are told otherwise, assume that you should use personal pronouns.

2   It uses language that is descriptive and specific to help the reader follow your link to the research. In the following example, for instance, fear can be shown in a way that suggests the uncertainty lying behind it:

> Mishel and Braden (1988) define uncertainty in illness as the inability to determine the meaning of illness related events, assign definite values to projects and/or accurately predict outcomes. Geeta expressed this when she pointed to a skyscraper overlooking her window and said, 'I feel like I have been chased to the top of that tall building, jumping down will lead to my death and returning means confronting my aggressors.' Here she depicts how her idea of a normal life has been replaced with fear, apprehension, complexity and uncertainty about what the future holds.

Reflective writing exercises

Here are some exercises you can do to improve your reflective abilities and writing skills. They all involve very intense and often very freeform writing activities, and can be a great deal of fun.

Personal journals

'Journal' comes from the French *jour*, which means 'day'. The idea is to write a little bit every day, even just a few minutes, to record what happened during your day and what you think or feel about it. A journal is a cumulative form of writing, unlike a research paper where you set aside a certain number of days to work on it and then it's done. Keeping a personal journal is 'one way of discovering sequence in experience, of stumbling upon cause and effect in the happenings of a writer's own life ... Connections slowly emerge ... Experiences ... connect and are identified as a larger shape' (Welty, 1984, cited in Kobert, 1995, p. 140). And the act of writing a little every day develops your writing skills – you will notice the difference within just a few weeks. Be aware, however, that keeping a journal is not always easy. There will be times when you have to force yourself to write, which will raise negative emotions and stifle creativity. At other times, you will miss a day (or days) because you are too busy and/or tired to write, and will feel guilty. Write as often as you can, especially if you have experienced some difficult situation to which you have had a strong emotional reaction. Conversely, it is important to capture those experiences which have been particularly inspiring or uplifting. But always make sure that you not only describe what has happened to you and what you felt about it, but that you also include some critical reflection on the issues raised by your experiences.

Freewriting

'Freewriting' refers to any writing process involving free association around a topic or question. It is a good exercise to engage in when you have done a little reading toward an assignment and want to start the writing process. Freewriting allows you to write without having to know what you want to say. It means not pausing to amend or even think about sentence structure or writing paragraphs, or even the quality of your words and ideas. In fact, don't think you need to write in a linear fashion at all, or fill the page from top to bottom. Write anywhere on the paper you wish, and feel free to add drawings if you are so inclined. Write for a predetermined length of time, perhaps five minutes when you start freewriting and increasing to ten or 15 minutes as you become more proficient.

Inkshedding

Unlike the very private process of freewriting, inkshedding is public, done together with a group. To 'inkshed' is to shed ink – that is, to freewrite while focused on a particular topic, question, reading, or class/tutorial decided upon by the group. To inkshed, you don't have to think hard – without stopping, just write whatever words come out about the topic, as points, sentences and/or paragraphs. After ten or 15 minutes, the group begins exchanging inksheds and responding to them – bracketing or underlining words/ points they think are important, adding marginal comments or expansions of the idea. When everyone has had a chance to respond to everyone else's, the papers come home to their writers, and the session ends with an open discussion of the inksheds (see Russ Hunt, *What is Inkshedding?* www. stthomasu.ca~hunt/dialogic/whatshed.htm).

Poetry

Poetry compresses meaning and human experience into individual words.

Writing poetry can be a free-form, free-associative experience, or it can be as formally composed as haiku or a sonnet. Either way, poetry forces the writer into deep reflection on the meanings, emotional impact and rhythm of every word chosen.

NARRATIVE AND THE ILLNESS EXPERIENCE

Nursing theorists study what they call the 'lived experience' and speak of the 'lived' body as opposed to the 'object' body. The object body is just that, a physical object in need of medical repair. Consider, for example, the case of a body with a malignant breast tumour. A surgeon can lay open the breast, remove the tumour, and stitch the body back together again. Barring complications, this is a process that doesn't vary much from one body to the next. But that object body is also a lived body – a woman with a life prior to the cancer that was disrupted by her diagnosis, who now suffers physically and emotionally with the many steps of the disease and treatment trajectory, who has hopes and fears for the future. To take another example, consider the case of a pregnant woman. Is her pregnancy just a medical condition to be monitored and managed to a successful outcome? What about the factors in her life that constitute the experience of pregnancy for her – her social supports (or lack of them), her preparedness (or not) for motherhood, any other children she may have, her financial situation, her education, and so on. All of these aspects of her life will impact on her ability to have a healthy pregnancy and a successful birth experience, as well as to give her newborn the best possible start in life.

'Narrative' writing, telling our stories and those of our patients, is one of our best methods of capturing the lived experience of illness and recovery. In the following example of a narrative section from a fourth year nursing student's reflective paper, notice a few things about the way she tells her patient's story:

1   She is clear and concise in describing her patient's pathophysiology and her nursing interventions.
2   She then lets J.D. speak for herself.
3   Finally she describes how the experience changed her perspective on what it means to live with a disability, and she begins to question her own nursing practices:

J.D. is a 15-year-old teenage girl whom I cared for at The Children's Center for the last two weeks. She used to be a healthy child and an excellent student who enjoyed reading, playing on the computer and hanging out with her friends. However, an unexpected disease has disrupted her normal life.

About six months ago, J.D. was diagnosed in hospital with Transverse Myelitis (TM), which is a neurological syndrome caused by inflammation of the spinal cord. Since the spinal cord carries motor nerve fibers to the limbs and trunk and sensory fibers from the body back to the brain, inflammation within the spinal cord interrupts these pathways and causes the common presenting symptoms of TM. These include limb weakness, sensory disturbance, bowel and bladder dysfunction, back pain and radicular pain.

J.D. has presented most of the symptoms mentioned above. Because her spinal cord has been damaged up to the level of T5, J.D. became wheelchair bound due to her inability to move her legs. She also developed bowel and bladder dysfunction. Two months ago, when her condition was stable, she was discharged from hospital to The Children's Centre for rehabilitation and habilitation.

According to J.D.'s daily routine, she goes to the school on site in both morning and afternoon. She also needs to have her urine catheterization done every four hours because of her incontinence. Overall she is pretty dependent in terms of self-care. Therefore, considering time for her school and physical therapies, I need to plan my day carefully to get all her nursing care done in a limited time. One morning when I walked into J.D.'s room and started to perform morning care for her as usual, I saw she was sad and tearful. And then she asked me, 'do you think I will be able to move? I just want to walk to do things that I used to do before. I don't care if I have sensation, but just walk.' I was a little bit shocked by her strong reaction to being in a wheelchair. Even though I have noticed that her mood seemed to be low, I have never offered her or her mother a chance to talk about their feelings and concerns. I have focused only on providing her with good care to make her physically comfortable. At that moment, I realized that I have missed the most important aspect of nursing care – caring for patients' emotional and psychosocial well-being and understanding their experience of disability. I started to wonder about what it meant to be confined to a wheelchair and what it would mean to me. Moreover, I realized that my nursing care was limited to my patients without including their families.

JOURNAL WRITING: LINKING REFLECTION TO THEORY AND PRACTICE

In a classic article on journal writing, Toby Fulwiler (1982) writes:

> Journals might be looked at as part of a continuum including diaries and class notebooks: while diaries record the private thought and experience of the writer, class notebooks record the public thought and presentation of the teacher. The journal is somewhere between the two. Like the diary, the journal is written in the first person about ideas important to the writer; like the class notebook, the journal may focus on academic subjects the writer wishes to examine. (p. 17)

The journal offers a place to explore the personal side of nursing, and link your experiences to the theory emerging from readings, lectures and tutorial discussions. By asking you to explore your reactions to personal and professional experiences in light of the theory emerging from readings, lecture and class discussions, journal writing allows you to step back from your actions and move beyond the immediacy of a particular situation into a larger understanding of your practice and the profession.

Journal writing may also be a requirement of your clinical practicum. As you work with a preceptor, you may be asked to maintain a journal on your activities and learning in the clinical/practice setting. This journal will be a valuable source of communication between you and your clinical instructor as well as a tool to assist you in reflecting on your clinical experiences. For faculty, the journal presents an opportunity to dialogue with individual students to increase their understanding of them as learners, nurses, and people. Journals should be written on a weekly basis and may be reviewed by your instructor as frequently as every week, or may form a portfolio to be submitted once or twice a term.

How to structure a journal entry

The following questions to help you structure a journal entry are based on a classic list suggested by Holborn (1988, p. 206) as a way to reach a deeper understanding of experiences:

1 Describe the details of the event and your feelings about it. Include as much detail as you need to tell your story as it happened. Ask yourself, 'What really happened? Why was it important to me?'

2 Analyze the event. Ask yourself, 'What were the significant elements of this situation? How did it affect my behaviour, feelings and attitudes? Did it challenge my beliefs or thinking? How did my behaviour affect the situation (for better or worse)? How is this situation like others I have experienced? Are there any patterns in the way I usually react to these situations?'

3 Analyze the event in terms of theoretical perspectives. Ask yourself, 'Is there a theoretical perspective that provides a way for me to understand what happened to me?'

4 Describe what you have learned from this incident. Ask yourself, 'How does this incident affect me? What do I know now that I didn't know before? Has this incident affected my beliefs, my values or the way I think about myself and others?'

5 Devise a plan of action for the future. Ask yourself, 'How will I apply what I have learned in another situation? Does theory or research give me a different point of view that can guide my future practice?'

Final example

In this excerpt from the same paper we read above, the writer delves into the meaning of her experience caring for J.D., what theoretical perspectives have to offer, and how she plans to change her practice based on her new insights:

Reading articles about disability theory reinforces for me that any social issues surrounding a patient's disability need to be addressed. From the perspective of the medical model, disability is considered a personal tragedy and a physical deficit. When I cared for J.D., I focused more on her functional limitations than her abilities to accomplish things. In the article on Disability and the Body, however, Hughes (1997) argues that 'disability should be understood not as a corporeal deficit but in terms of the ways in which social structure excludes and oppresses disabled people.' By reading these articles, my view of disability has been changed. The medical model sees part of the problem, but the social model allows me to see the problem in a broader way. When working with children living with disabilities, I need to be aware of social barriers that are imposed on these children. For example, J.D. has not seen her friends for months because nobody has called her back or visited her since she was hospitalized. Loss of peer contact has made her sad and depressed. Wendell (1998) states that "disabled people are 'other' to able-bodied people and the consequences are socially, economically and psychologically oppressive to the disabled" (p. 271). Based on the above statement, I believe that J.D. is no longer accepted into her peer group because her disability made her different from her peers. People fear being the 'other' and also don't know how to deal with it. I'm also left with an uncomfortable question about myself – have I focused so much on her physical care because I too have been seeing her as 'other'?

J.D. has been isolated from her former life as an active, happy teenager. She feels confined not just to a wheelchair but to a new life that is lonely. She needs not just physical treatment but also psychosocial support, from her friends and from me as her nurse.

For further reading

Darbyshire, P. (1995). Lessons from literature: Caring, interpretation, and dialogue. *Journal of Nursing Education 34*(5), 211–216.

Fulwiler, T. (1982). The personal connection: Journal writing across the curriculum (pp. 15–30). In T. Fulwiler & A. Young (Eds.), *Language connections: Writing and reading across the curriculum.* Urbana, IL: National Council of Teachers of English.

Hecker, T., Amon, J., & Nickoli, E. *Reflective writing in nursing.* Retrieved August 18, 2000 from http://www.cariboo.bc.ca/Disciplines/eng309/nursing/nursing.htm

Holborn, P. (1988). Becoming a reflective practitioner. In P. Holborn, M. Wideen, & I. Andrews (Eds.), *Becoming a teacher* (pp. 203–206). Toronto, ON: Kagan & Woo.

Kobert, L.J. (1995). In our own voice: Journaling as a teaching/learning technique for nurses. *Journal of Nursing Education 34*(3), 140–142.

Lauterbach, S. S., & Becker, P. H. (1996). Caring for self: Becoming a self-reflective nurse. *Holistic Nursing Practice 10*(2), 57–68.

Nehls, N. (1995). Narrative pedagogy: Rethinking nursing education. *Journal of Nursing Education 34*(5), 204–210.

HOW TO WRITE COURSE PAPERS: *12* SAMPLES OF STUDENT WRITING

> ## OVERVIEW
>
> - What are markers looking for?
> - Sample paper 1: writing that integrates theory
> - Sample paper 2: writing a case study
> - Sample paper 3: writing about pathophysiology

WHAT ARE MARKERS LOOKING FOR?

You can use this checklist to help you preview how an instructor might read your work – or ask a fellow student to 'mark' your paper using it. The four areas – topic, ideas, organization, and expression – are the ones markers concentrate on in assigning grades.

You don't have to assign yourself grades, though they're included if you wish to. If you do use them, use 'C' as your starting point (that is, have the expectation that you've written an adequate paper), and move up or down from there.

Topic

- Is there a clear definition of what the central topic, problem or issue is? Is it described clearly and precisely?
- Is the topic sufficiently narrowed or broadened such that it can be dealt with fully in the assigned length?
- Is there a clear rationale for analyzing or discussing this topic? Have you established why your topic is important, and to whom?
- Is there a clear thesis or perspective on the topic (e.g., not just 'what,' but 'what about it')?
- Does the paper stick to the topic, or does it sometimes wander to other topics?

Ideas

- Is the content appropriate to the topic or question posed? Is the level of detail appropriate to how broad or narrow the paper's focus is?
- Is there a good balance between ideas and evidence, or evidence and interpretation?
- Have you understood and applied the literature and the theories, or have you merely read and regurgitated them? Have you explained the ideas and findings of others in your own words? Have you described their strengths and weaknesses?
- Have you shown which approaches have been taken to your topic or problem? Do you show awareness of problematic or controversial elements, awareness of potential objections or alternative approaches?
- Are you too general, too descriptive, too full of generalizations that can't be supported? Are your ideas clichéd, or repetitious?
- Does the argument (ideas + evidence) made in the body connect to the topic, and does it lead logically and inevitably to your conclusion(s)?

Organization and structure

- Are there clearly defined sections in the paper that correspond to the particular requirements of the assignment? If headings are used, are they used logically?
- Does the introduction define the issue, state a rationale, and indicate a focus for your discussion/analysis?
- Does each paragraph in the body address a distinct idea, or contribute to the development of the distinct idea of its section? Is there unnecessary repetition?
- Does the conclusion merely restate the topic or thesis, or does it offer a genuine conclusion?
- The three principles of effective organization: does the paper as a whole, each section, each paragraph, and each sentence have:
  o **unity** (deals with one idea);
  o **coherence** (moves smoothly and logically); and
  o **emphasis** (important points strategically placed)?
- If there is an abstract, is it accurate, concise, self-contained, and readable?

Expression

- Is the writing style concise, direct, and interesting?
- Is there a good variety of sentence lengths and types?
- Is the tone appropriate?

- o   scientific: neutral;
- o   reflective: personal, creative, emotional, narrative.
- Are technical and scientific terms used correctly and consistently?
- Is the non-technical diction appropriate: good, varied vocabulary; precision in word choice; clear and simple over long and Latinate (e.g., 'ask for' vs. 'solicit')?
- Are there errors in 'mechanics': grammar, punctuation, usage, spelling?
- Are the citation, referencing and formatting complete and accurate?

In the following sections, a number of sample student papers are reproduced to demonstrate the structures and expectations of particular types of writing commonly asked for in nursing programs.

SAMPLE PAPER 1: WRITING THAT INTEGRATES THEORY

What is theory?

A 'theory' is a set of ideas used in order to contemplate something in order to explain or understand it. In contrast, 'practice' refers to the idea of taking action. In the health professions, we may theorize about what it means to be 'healthy' or 'sick' or have a 'good quality of life'. At the same time, we put our theory into practice by offering prenatal classes, performing nursing assessments and interventions, or engaging in palliative care to help our patients die with dignity. See Chapter 8 for a description of macro-level and middle-range theories used in the nursing literature. You can consider 'theoretical perspective', 'theoretical lens' and 'theoretical framework' to be synonymous terms that refer to the theory a writer is using.

Another important term in reading and writing about theory is 'concept'. It is perhaps best described by Green and Thorogood (2004):

> 'Concepts' are the building blocks of theory, the 'high-level' or abstract terms in which we frame our understanding of health. These refer to macro-theoretical constructs . . ., such as 'inequality', 'globalization', 'power', but also the middle-range theories in which our research questions are usually embedded. Here, concepts such as 'lifestyle', 'medical autonomy' or 'compliance' may be used as part of the common stock of knowledge within a particular discipline, but carry within them a set of (often implicit) assumptions. (p. 30)

How to write about theory

Chapter 3 talked about the 'front-end loaded' nature of the iterative writing process. For no type of writing is this more true than it is for writing about theory where words and concepts are multidimensional/multilayered. Before you can write about theory, you need to spend time thinking about it.

When you are in the active reading and brainstorming stage, trying to understand the theory you are reading about, it is very helpful to do a 'concept analysis' (Walker & Avant, 1983). Concept analysis is a strategy for extracting the defining characteristics of a concept by analyzing your course materials and your readings from the literature. Extracting these characteristics allows you to decide which phenomena are good examples of the concept and which are not. The process is similar to establishing criteria for a differential diagnosis: by clearly defining the criteria for a diagnosis, it becomes possible to name a specific condition as differentiated from another similar or related one. There are no rules for accomplishing a concept analysis: the process ranges from a formal linguistic exercise (Walker & Avant, 1983) used by nurse researchers to the brainstorming technique recommended here.

As part of your active reading process, highlight words or phrases that describe characteristics of the concept and make a list of them. Assign especial importance to the ones that recur over and over. This list of characteristics is called the 'defining attributes' (Walker & Avant, 1983) of a concept.

Many assignments that ask you to write about theory will ask you to use your personal experience to illuminate the theory, or vice versa. Thus, the next step in the brainstorming process is to link the attributes to a model case within your own experience or the readings. In the model case, seek out what are called 'empirical referents' for the concept. An empirical referent is a phenomenon in the real world that confirms that the concept is occurring. For example, in the sample paper below, 'take a deep loud breath' is an empirical referent for the concept of uncertainty. Describing these empirical referents helps to link theory to the real world of nursing and midwifery practice.

You will find on reflection that your model case fits with the characteristics and defining attributes in one of these ways identified by Walker and Avant (1983):

- the case is a 'real life' example of the use of the concept which includes *all* the defining attributes;
- a borderline case which contains *some* but not all of the attributes;
- a related case which is *similar* but doesn't contain the defining attributes;
- a contrary case which is a clear example of '*not-the-concept*';
- an illegitimate case which uses the concept term *improperly*.

Clearly, you will reject any experience that is neither a real-life nor a borderline model case and look for another that exemplifies the theory better.

For further reading

Green, J. & Thurgood, N. (2004). *Qualitative methods for health research*. London. Sage.
Walker, L.O. & Avant, K.C. (1983) *Strategies for theory construction in nursing*. Norwalk, CT: Appleton-Century-Crofts.

The sample paper by TH that is presented here discusses the concept of 'uncertainty in illness' using the real life example of one of her patients. It was written for a course in Nursing Issues in Neuroscience and Trauma. It received a grade of A, or First Class Honours, and the marker commented: 'Good flow, well structured, well written' of the paper, and that 'Theories from uncertainty are well understood and applied appropriately to this case study.' The paper can be deconstructed into four sections: introduction, first antecedent of uncertainty, second antecedent of uncertainty, and conclusion.

Antecedents of uncertainty in illness

by T_____H_____

Section one: introduction

[Note 1] During my neurological placement, I cared for a 44-year-old female, 'Geeta', who is a recent immigrant from India. She was admitted for left sided weakness and numbness of tongue with occasional vomiting. She had a supportive family which consisted of her husband and two children. I was amazed at the bond and love they shared. Occasionally, as I went in to care for Geeta, I heard them talk about their challenging experiences here in Canada and would jokingly blame Geeta for initiating the immigration process. They laughed and made statements like 'Canada, yours to discover.' To them, their mother's symptoms were just one of the usual issues that women of her age have and this admission was just a routine checkup. They were hopeful she would soon be back with them home so they could continue their 'discovery'; until the sudden diagnosis of metastatic melanoma was made on their mother. They were all devastated and consumed by the sudden turn of events. Being new immigrants, coupled with this sudden diagnosis of a life-altering and potentially life-threatening cancer, presented a doubly-stressful situation for both the patient and her family. [Note 2] Being a mother and a recent immigrant, I found this situation very challenging because I could relate to it. [Note 3] This paper will seek to examine this clinical case using the concept of patient uncertainty to highlight how my understanding was deepened by the multiple challenges that Geeta and her family were faced with in the diagnosis of her cancerous tumours.

[Note 4] During this clinical encounter with Geeta, the concept of the antecedent of uncertainty as studied by Mishel and Braden (1988) and Wallace (2005) provided me with a sound understanding of how Geeta dealt with her new diagnosis. The study by Mishel and Braden revealed that the presence of uncertainty did not develop spontaneously in their participants, but was influenced by antecedents in three categories of variables: stimuli frame (form, composition and structure of the stimuli contained in illness and treatment related events) and structure providers (resources available to assist the person in the interpretation of the stimuli frame). The study identified symptom pattern and event familiarity as sub-concepts of stimuli frame, and education, social support and credible authority as sub-concepts of structure providers that have the greatest influence on lowering the level of uncertainty.

I hope to illustrate, as [Note 5] McCormick (2002) argues, that uncertainty is a multidimensional concept and a major component of the illness experience that can dramatically affect psychosocial adaptation and outcomes of disease states. [Note 6] To do so, I will use the stimuli frame concepts of symptom pattern and event familiarity, and the structure provider concepts of education and credible authority discussed by Mishel and Braden (1988) and Wallace (2005) to analyze this clinical situation.

Section two: first antecedent of uncertainty (symptom pattern and event familiarity)

[Note 7] Mishel and Braden (1988) define uncertainty in illness as the inability to determine the meaning of illness related events, assign definite values to projects and events, and/or accurately predict outcomes. Geeta expressed this when she pointed to a skyscraper overlooking her window and said, 'I feel like I have been chased to the top of that tall building, jumping down will lead to my death and returning means confronting my aggressors.' Here she depicts how her idea of a normal life has been replaced with [Note 8] fear, apprehension, complexity and uncertainty about what the future holds.

An overt, recurrent symptom presents a [Note 9] symptom pattern that facilitates deriving meaning and understanding for an individual regarding an illness state (Neville, 2003). A symptom pattern can lead to less uncertainty and less ambiguity about the state of illness (Mishel & Braden, 1988). [Note 10] In this clinical situation, the sudden throbbing headache accompanied by severe weakness and vomiting Geeta was experiencing was a revelation of a diseased body and an indication of an illness state. Although she was given medication which temporarily alleviated the symptoms, she did not gain control of the situation. Her uncertainty worsened. This can be attributed to the background meaning brain tumours and their negative prognosis have for her. To her, a diagnosis of brain tumour was a death sentence. [Note 11] In my bid to console her and instill hope, I said to her, 'Everything is going to be fine.' Reflecting on this situation, I recognize that my response was unguarded and I created false hope by overplaying the likelihood of complete recovery. Rather, I could have engaged her on what the new diagnosis meant to her. Based on her response, we could have both explored options available to her, and how she could take advantage of them to gain mastery over her situation. This I believe would have helped create and sustain a sense of inner tranquility in the face of difficult realities.

[Note 12] . . . .

Section three: second antecedent of uncertainty

From Mishel and Braden (1988) I can see that structure providers, especially [Note 13] education and credible authority, are the resources available that could assist Geeta and her family to interpret these overwhelming encounters.

Wallace (2005), who expanded on Mishel and Braden's work, found a positive correlation between education and a person's level of uncertainty. He argued that education broadened and deepened the patients' knowledge base, making interpretation of their symptoms better, thereby enhancing their familiarity of events. Furthermore, education made assimilation of information easier compared to less education which required more time for explanation, thus prolonging uncertainty. Education here was measured in number of school years. [Note 14] This is directly applicable to this case in question; being a high school graduate and a recent immigrant, Geeta would most likely be less educated than many other cancer patients. She would likely have language barriers and trouble understanding specific facts about her diagnosis as well as challenges navigating the healthcare system. As a new immigrant, there might be areas where she may be lacking in adequate healthcare coverage as well as social and economic factors, making her uncertainty even more apparent. In anguish, she would quickly turn to look at her husband and ask, 'what did they say?' after every visit by a consultant. [Note 15] As a novice nurse, this did not clue me in. I assumed that she was just not paying attention or at worst that her cognitive capacity had been impaired by her medications (Mishel & Braden, 1988) which mostly made her drowsy. In my effort to help, I repeated exactly what was said in the same words and medical jargon. She would then gaze at me for a while and take a deep loud breath. Looking back, I could have been more helpful in reducing her anxiety by explaining all information in simple terms to her. I could have also advocated for her by making other healthcare professionals aware of her challenges and the need to avoid complicated medical jargon.

[Note 16] . . . .

Section four: conclusion

[Note 17] Early in diagnosis, a high level of uncertainty exists regarding the progression and severity of the illness as well as extent of bodily areas of involvement (Neville, 2003). As nurses, we need to pay attention to our patient's real or potential fears and concerns regarding uncertainty that ensues with illness. As reiterated by Neville (2003), this is an important aspect of providing comprehensive care. [Note 18] It is also clear that the patient's family will need to be involved to help the patient cope; this was the greatest insight I gained in reading the theoretical foundations that will help guide Geeta's care. As a result, the treatment plan for Geeta must include emotional and physical support for her family members. It is clear from Wallace (2005) that family members of cancer patients experience personal struggles coping with their own feelings during their loved one's illness, yet they feel they need to display compassion towards the patient and 'stay strong' for them. [Note 19] For my future practice, I will establish connection with patients and families as a source for information and therapeutic support; I will assist them to find meaning by providing cues about physical aspects and efficacy of treatments, and expectations about outcomes; I will keep them informed about protocols, scheduling, effect of treatments and prognosis; and prepare them for an event or treatment, by providing both sensory and cognitive information. I believe this will allay the feelings of assault and disruption of their daily lives dealt to them by the diagnosis. In addition, I will always apply theoretical concepts in my care of patients, as this case has shown that theory is an essential part of the nursing profession.

Notes on sample paper 1

1 This paragraph gives a) a description of the case that includes both the diagnosis and the family.
2 b) Similarities between Geeta and TH's social location as mothers and recent immigrants.
3 c) Identifies the purpose of the paper.
4 This paragraph introduces the concept of uncertainty and identifies three categories of antecedents of uncertainty plus three sub-concepts.
5 McCormick's article performs a formal concept analysis of 'uncertainty'. When shaping her own understanding of the concept, TH would have read that 'characteristics of the illness situation – ambiguity, vagueness, unpredictability, unfamiliarity, inconsistency, and lack of information – underlie the process of uncertainty'.
6 Here, TH identifies the two antecedents of uncertainty that will be applied to the case: stimuli frame and structure providers.
7 The introductory paragraph in the second section of the paper defines uncertainty and uses the case to illustrate the definition.
8 Here TH identifies four more characteristics of uncertainty and relates them to her patient.
9 Introduces the first concept (symptom pattern) and defines it.
10 Relates the concept to the clinical situation.
11 TH integrates personal reflection on her role as Geeta's nurse.
12 TH's next paragraph, on event familiarity, is not included here.
13 Announces the two structure providers the section will discuss.

14 TH applies the structure provider, education, to Geeta's case.
15 TH shows a great deal of insight in this section into a common frustration faced by patients when health professionals speak in medical jargon.
16 Two paragraphs follow. The first discusses the role of the nurse as a 'credible authority' for information and advocacy; the second discusses some contrasting findings about uncertainty in the studies by Mishel & Braden and Wallace.
17 The concluding paragraph (a) relates the concept of uncertainty to nursing practice;
18 (b) emphasizes the importance of family in planning care to reduce uncertainty;
19 (c) concludes by summarizing specific ways TH plans to reduce uncertainty for her patients in her future practice. All of these are described more fully in the body of the paper.

SAMPLE PAPER 2: WRITING A CASE STUDY

A case study is a type of assignment that requires multiple forms of writing: narrative (telling the story of the patient, the family, and the role of the nurse), pathophysiology (describing the medical and nursing assessments and interventions), reflective writing (describing the nurse's engagement in family-centred care), and evidence-based practice (using the research literature to support the diagnosis and interventions).

This sample of a case study received first-class honours. The strengths of the paper noted by the marker are that a) the care of the baby and her family is described and explained in detail, and b) every step of the care is backed up by support from research and standards of care.

Introduction

[Note 1] The following case study explores the acute illness bronchiolitis, defining its disease process, gaining insight into the epidemiological data, and providing pathophysiological information relating to the infection. This case study also emphasises the importance of Family Centred Care, and the way in which the nurse should work not only with the child, but also with their families (Franck and Callery 2004). The aspect of Family Centred Care will be integrated throughout this case study but will be discussed in full within the designated section. According to Young et al. (2006: 7) the practice of the nurse must be adapted so as to 'include the family to the greatest extent', whilst always ensuring that the needs of the child are the leading point in care. In order to do this, a five-week-old baby girl (suffering with bronchiolitis) and her family have been selected, and the care they received during their stay at hospital will be focused upon. The NMC (2008: 1) guidelines on confidentiality state that 'everyone has the right to respect for his private and family life, his home and his correspondence' and forbids the disclosure of personal information outside the clinical setting. Thus, in order to protect the privacy of the baby girl and her family, she will be referred to as 'Holly'. [Note 2]

[Note 3] Holly was admitted to the ward following a GP referral, and her parents stated that she had been unwell for 48 hours. Holly presented with a history of nasal secretions and a cough, and it was reported that her feeds had been taking longer than normal. No diarrhoea or vomiting had occurred, but Holly had been very unsettled the previous night. The GP had documented that Holly had been short of breath and tachypneic during his assessment.

Holly entered the ward at 12.30pm, and was still short of breath on arrival. Her observations were fairly stable (in accordance with the RCN 2007 'Standards for assessing, measuring and monitoring vital signs in infants'), with a temperature of 37.6 degrees, a respiratory rate of 48 breaths per minute, and a capillary refill time of 2 seconds. Her apex beat, however – at 173 – was on the higher side of normality for her age, while her oxygen saturation levels were dipping to 95%. Holly's weight was recorded at 2.95kg. As bronchiolitis was suspected, Holly was immediately isolated to prevent the spread of infection. The doctors at the hospital prescribed Holly with Saline Nasal Drops PRN, 60mg of Paracetamol QDS and 15mg of Ibuprofen 8 hourly. However, it is important to note that NICE (2007) guidelines on 'Feverish Illness in Children' state that the latter should only be given if the child fails to respond to the first given agent, as opposed to both being prescribed for routine administration. The BNFC (2006) also specifies that Ibuprofen should not be prescribed to children under the age of 3 months, and is not licensed for children weighing less than 5kg, while Paracetamol should be provided 8 hourly for an infant of Holly's age.

On the night of her admission, Holly's oxygen saturation levels dropped to 88–92%, leading to 0.2 litres of oxygen being provided via a nasal cannula. At this point, I noticed that Holly was 'head bobbing' and the doctors were informed. Following a review, it was also stated that Holly had intercostal recession, and that her vital signs were to be observed and recorded hourly for six hours (0000 to 0600) in order to monitor any changes. Holly's Nasopharyngeal Aspirate results confirmed that she was RSV positive. Despite the fact that Holly's feeds of SMA Gold had been calculated (in accordance with her weight) at 295ml in 24 hours, her oral intake had reduced significantly. For this reason, a nasogastric tube was passed and Holly received 24mls of milk 2 hourly to begin. As Holly tolerated her feeds well, she was later able to receive 36mls 3 hourly, and 49mls 4 hourly the following day.

Three days after admission, Holly showed substantial signs of improvement and was taking oral feeds once more. As a result of this, her nasogastric tube was removed. She was also weaned from oxygen. 24 hours later, Holly and her family were prepared for discharge as she was able to maintain her saturations at a satisfactory level in air.

[Note 4] Holly and her family were selected for this case study because I spent a large amount of time with her and was constantly involved in her care, giving me the opportunity to get to know her and her family well. Because of this, I was able to provide care for her that I did not provide for most other children. For example, I had the opportunity to feed Holly both nasogastrically and orally on numerous occasions, as well as to bath her with the help of a Healthcare Assistant. Under these circumstances, I was able to learn the importance of ensuring that an infant at risk of de-saturating is kept in an upright position, 'reducing pressure on the diaphragm in order to ease abdominal breathing' (Lambert 2004: 29). According to Thoyre and Carlson (2003), attention must also be paid to any changes in sounds of breathing in these situations in order to determine whether or not intervention is needed to prevent oxygen decline. The rate, rhythm, frequency and depth of breathing should additionally be monitored in order to detect signs of deterioration (Trim 2005).

I was also personally able to educate Holly's parents with their infant's care. For example, her mother reported that Holly's nose appeared to be 'blocked' and so I administered Saline Nasal Drops, explaining how to do so and leaving some behind in the cubicle in order for her mother to use later that day if needed. She was also concerned that as her baby was unwell, 'picking her up' would cause a deterioration in Holly's condition. I re-assured her that she would still be able to lift and hold Holly, as an infant crying may simply mean that they want to be comforted, and that holding Holly in a semi-upright position (as discussed above by Lambert 2004) would in fact be beneficial to her condition.

Additionally, I was able to monitor Holly's vital signs by day and by night, observing the difference in clinical symptoms depending on the time. During a night shift, it was me personally who noticed that Holly was 'head bobbing', a sign of respiratory distress (Patient UK, 2008), and informed the doctors of my concerns that her breathing had become irregular. Following review, the doctors reported that Holly was still exhibiting signs of intercostal recession, prescribed her with oxygen, and asked me to perform hourly observations until improvement was shown.

The final (and most important) reason for selecting Holly is the fact that bronchiolitis is a common respiratory infection and it is estimated that a third of infants in the UK develop bronchiolitis in their first year of life (NHS Choices 2010). This case study will therefore provide the opportunity to gain a wide and useful insight into bronchiolitis, an infection which will often be encountered in future work on paediatric medical wards.

. . . . [Note 5]

Assessment & Nursing Intervention [Note 6]

With regards to assessment, the Nursing and Midwifery Council (2008) describes the need for holism, and the importance of considering the 'psychological, social and spiritual needs of the patient' as well as the physical. They also explore the need for constant re-assessment, as in order to intervene accurately and consistently, the healthcare professional should perform regular observations. It is therefore essential that, on beginning the assessment of the patient and their family, all areas relating to health, lifestyle and welfare are constantly observed and re-assessed as the condition of the patient dicta... The assessment undertaken should be extensive, as well as precise and methodical (NHS Blackpool Primary Care Trust 2007).

[Note 7] The Roper, Logan and Tierney 'Model of Nursing' (1980) is one which considers the patient 'as a whole' (Langford 2007), focusing on areas vital for maintaining life, as well as areas to improve the quality of living. For these reasons, this model will be used in order to discuss the way in which the bronchiolitis patient should be assessed, and examples of Holly's care will be mentioned, as the 'Activities of Living' were applied directly to her and her family.

An assessment should always begin by the nurse introducing him- or herself to the patient and their families, and (in turn) requesting that the names of the clients are shared (Pullen and Mathias 2010). Effective communication is crucial within the healthcare setting, as it can instantly provide reassurance towards the unknown and the opportunity to develop a nurse–patient rapport (Engel 2002). Children being admitted to hospital with bronchiolitis are likely to be very young (Gilbert 1999), so the majority of verbal communication undertaken will be between the nurse and the parents or guardians. However, in addition, communication can be non-verbal and attempting to soothe the distressed infant by touch can also have therapeutic effects (Roper et al. 2000). It is also vital for the nurse to listen intently to any information shared by the family, constantly re-enforcing that their participation in care is 'worthwhile' (Engel 2002: 8). Thorough and detailed communication should be implemented throughout the care of the child, and the parents or guardian of the infant should be updated in care planning at all times (Espezel and Canam 2003, Law et al. 2003).

. . . . [Note 8]

We must secondly consider the activity of 'Eating and Drinking'. Regular consumption of food and fluid provides the human body with energy (Roper et al. 2000). The energy produced subsequently ensures that growth, development and continuous cell activity are able to occur.

Infants suffering with respiratory distress may become exhausted, and it is for these reasons that SIGN (2006) discusses reduced oral intake as a prototypical clinical feature of bronchiolitis; stating that 'poor feeding' can be diagnosed if the infant is consuming less than 50% of his or her usual oral intake. A study undertaken by Unger and Cunningham (2008) showed that the majority (at 82%) of bronchiolitis patients presented with feeding difficulties on admission. This is a symptom which (as earlier discussed) was exhibited by Holly.

[Note 9] Infants are particularly susceptible to becoming dehydrated because water accounts for 75% of body weight at birth, as opposed to water accounting for 60% of body weight in adulthood. This, in addition to the infant having a larger surface area, a proportionally longer gastrointestinal tract and being unable to satisfy his or her own thirst would make them more prone to dehydration (Broom 2004). Symptoms that may indicate dehydration in the child include dry mucous membranes, reduced urine output and irritability. The dehydrated child may also have sunken eyes and a sunken fontanelle, as well as weight loss and an increasing pulse (NHS Choices 2009). It is therefore essential that the nurse calculates the required fluid intake for the child in accordance with their weight and (possibly with parental assistance) monitors and records this along with the fluid output; so to prevent dehydration at the earliest possible stage. Smaller, more frequent feeds may need to be considered if the infant is having problems feeding. However, if the baby (like Holly) continues to become intolerant to oral feeds, a nasogastric tube should be inserted, and nasogastric feeding commenced (SIGN 2006). In order to test that the nasogastric tube has been correctly positioned, the Medicines and Healthcare Products Regulatory Agency (2004) advised that aspiration and pH paper testing should be used before every feed (Taylor and Clemente 2005). Following insertion, the nurse must still continue to monitor fluid intake and output; adjusting the volume and frequency of the feeds as the condition of the infant dictates. When the infant is able to tolerate oral feeds once more, the nasogastric tube can be removed.

. . . . [Note 10]

[Note 11] To conclude, the nurse should take the points discussed into consideration whilst always remembering the importance of re-assessing and altering the care of the child as their condition dictates. Final 'Activities of Living' that would also be considered are 'Eliminating', 'Personal Cleansing' and 'Dressing' (Roper et al. 2000).

Family Centred Care [Note 12]

Family Centred Care can be defined as a concept in which the care of the child is interlinked with the care of the family, embracing their involvement and recognizing their central role (Smith, Coleman and Bradshaw 2006: 77).

Smith, Coleman and Bradshaw (2002) cited in Smith, Coleman and Bradshaw (2006: 80) developed a 'Practice Continuum Tool', designed for use within the clinical environment. The spectrum of the tool ranges from care being completely 'nurse-led' with no family involvement, to care being 'parent-led' with nurse consultation. Between these markers are 'nurse-led' care with 'family involvement', 'nurse-led' care with 'family participation' and an 'equal status', with a 'family partnership' in the care of the child.

During Holly's stay at hospital, her care consisted mostly of the nursing team taking the lead in management, with the family becoming involved in the provision of basic or routine procedures (such as hygiene, feeding and emotional support). Their reasoning for not partaking in further aspects of nursing care was that, as Holly (at 5 weeks old) was of such a young age, they were apprehensive about making a mistake and felt that the nursing team would be able to intervene and assist Holly with greater success. This however did alter at times; for example, with encouragement and education, Holly's mother was able to administer Saline Nasal Drops in order to clear the secretions from her infant's nose. As Smith et al. (2006: 80) state, families are encouraged to move in 'either direction at any time' on the continuum tool as their individual needs and dynamics dictate. Nurses should therefore be willing to adapt their practice constantly so to suit the needs of the family as and when they alter.

One example of a time when the nursing team offered to adapt their practice and take a complete lead in care in order to help the family was on the third night of Holly's stay. Holly's mother was epileptic, and expressed her concerns over the fact that she was most likely to suffer with a seizure when she was tired. She felt as if the stress of her new baby being admitted to hospital had left her feeling so anxious that she had been unable to sleep at all, and (as a result) was exhausted. As Diaz-Caneja et al. (2005) state, the admission of a child to hospital can be extremely distressing for the parent. The care team therefore offered to feed Holly and closely monitor her throughout the night so that some of the pressure was relieved from her mother, leaving her to sleep as she wished. It was agreed that, by doing this, Holly's mother would feel better the next day, be less likely to suffer with a seizure and would be able to provide improved care for her daughter with greater levels of energy.

. . . . [Note 13]

Conclusion [Note 14]

[Note 15] The aim of this case study was to explore the acute illness bronchiolitis, providing a pathophysiological definition and exploring the disease process. In order to complete this case study, the care of the five-week-old infant, 'Holly' and her family was focused upon. As Holly was suffering from bronchiolitis and was experiencing the problems above, a range of intervening procedures were provided to assist in stabilizing her condition. Despite the fact that most of the intervening procedures proved to be age appropriate and successful, research by Chandler (2001) suggests that the use of the head box may have proven to be more beneficial and comfortable than the chosen nasal prongs for the provision of oxygen therapy for a five-week-old baby. In reflection, this could have been suggested at the time of intervention and discussed in detail with the care team.

[Note 16] This case study also aimed to explore the concept of 'Family Centred Care', and the notion that the care of the family is equally important as the care of the ill child (Young et al. 2006). As Smith et al. (2006) stated, families within the healthcare setting can become as involved as they wish with the care of their child in hospital, depending on the individual family needs and dynamics (which can often alter day by day). The nursing team would therefore need to constantly adapt their practice to suit the changing needs of each family in their care (Franck and Callery 2004).

[Note 17] Reflecting on the Family Centred Care provided for Holly and her family, the nursing team were consistent in ensuring that their psychological and social needs were constantly met. As a result of this, a good rapport was established and negative emotions (such as anxiety and depression) were avoided as far as possible (Whiting 2006). The nursing team also worked well to ensure that any sibling rivalry was prevented (Dowle and Siddall 2006, Moules and Ramsay 2008).

The fact that the needs of the child and their family are constantly changing reinforces the importance of constant re-assessment within the healthcare setting (NMC 2008). To ensure that the needs of Holly and her family were met, the healthcare team thoroughly performed regular observations and updated her care planning as her condition or situation dictated.

[Note 18] To conclude, nurses must be flexible and efficient in the care of the bronchiolitis patient, and constantly adapt their practice to suit the ever-changing needs of the child and the family (Young et al. 2006, NMC 2008).

Notes on sample paper 2

1   The first paragraph immediately identifies what the paper is (case study) and then goes on to summarize its contents.
2   This is the correct way to introduce a pseudonym: put the name into quotation marks, single or double, the first time you give the name.
3   The next four paragraphs tell the story of Holly's three-day hospital admission. Included are her presenting symptoms, her medical and nursing care, and her discharge.

4   The next three paragraphs explain the reasons this case was selected and describe the many opportunities the writer had to care for Holly and her family.

5   The pathophysiology section of the paper follows but has been omitted here because a sample pathophysiology paper is given below.

6   This section discusses the first topic of the case study: Holly's bronchiolotis and how it is assessed and treated.

7   This paragraph identifies the model of nursing used in the case study, as well as the two topics that are covered: bronchiolitis and family-centred care.

8   The paper goes through four 'Activities of Living', relating each of these aspects of Roper et al.'s model to Holly's care. The first one, on performing an 'ABC assessment' (airway, breathing and circulation) is omitted.

9   Dehydration is explained, and every action the nurse should take is clearly described.

10   Two sections of 'Activities of Living' have been omitted: 'Maintaining a Safe Environment' and 'Controlling Body Temperature'.

11   A brief paragraph concludes the section by listing other activities the nurse should integrate into care.

12   This section covers the second topic of the case study: family-centred care.

13   Three other examples of family-centred care have been omitted, including a discussion of the family dynamics.

14   The conclusion summarizes everything that was discussed in the paper.

15   The first part of the conclusion summarizes the first topic of the case study: bronchiolitis.

16   The second part of the conclusion summarizes the second topic of the case study: family-centred care.

17   This paragraph and the next provide a summary reflection and overall evaluation of the quality of family-centred care in this case.

18   The final short paragraph brings the reader back to the two topics of the case study: the care of bronchiolitis and the care of the family.

SAMPLE PAPER 3: WRITING ABOUT PATHOPHYSIOLOGY

Pathophysiology writing represents evidence-based practice in action. The goal is to describe a case, evaluate potential diagnoses and treatments, and make recommendations for case management and follow-up. This sample paper by P.A. received a grade of A/First class honours.

Acute exacerbated chronic obstructive pulmonary disease: pathophysiology and pharmacotherapeutics [Note 1]

by P.A.

Introduction [Note 2]

[Note 3] The intent of this paper is to examine the medical condition of my acute care patient who I will refer to as PC. On March 21, 2011, PC, an 89-year-old male who was diagnosed with Chronic Obstructive Pulmonary Disease (COPD) in 1999, was admitted to hospital after a week of experiencing some cold symptoms, fever, persistent cough with purulent sputum production and progressive shortness of breath (SOB) which was unrelieved by the use of his puffers. Examination prior to admission revealed rapid and shallow respirations of 48 breaths per minute; with prolonged expiratory phase plus grunting and pursed lip breathing. PC's oxygen saturation was 85% on 2L oxygen via nasal prongs. His breath sounds were diminished bilaterally during inspiration with expiratory wheezing upon auscultation. Percussion of his chest revealed dullness. He had a fever with oral temperature of 38.1 degree Celsius, pulse rate of 138 beats per minute and +4 pitting edema on both legs from knee downwards. His demeanour showed signs of distress and anxiety. His admitting diagnosis was Acute Exacerbated Chronic Obstructive Pulmonary Disease (AECOPD).

[Note 4] In this paper, I will review the pathophysiological background of PC's obstructive airway disease, and explore any interrelatedness to his previous lifestyle of smoking as well as any systemic effects it has had on his other medical conditions. I will also examine the pharmacotherapeutic interventions to relieve his illness and symptoms, specifically looking at their mechanism of action, any actual or potential interactions, and relating this back to the pathophysiology of PC's condition, highlighting any possible side effects. Lastly, I will address the nursing implications for monitoring PC during the course of his illness and discuss any future needs or follow-up related to his pathophysiological and pharmacological needs.

Demographics [Note 5]

PC is an 89-year-old male, married with three children and six grandchildren. He is 6 feet 3 inches and weighs 76kg (standing scale), indicating a weight loss of 4kg from his last visit to Emergency earlier on in the week. His previous health history includes congestive heart failure (CHF) with IV LV, pulmonary hypertension, myocardial infarction with CABG, hypertension, dyslipidemia and atrial fibrillation. PC, a staunch Anglican, is a third generation Canadian born to an Anglican clergyman. PC worked as an investment banker on Wall Street and later at the Bank of Montreal until his retirement. PC has had a long history of smoking, with approximately 55 pack years. PC, who is at the integrity and despair stage in Erikson's developmental model, talks happily about the good times he has had in life, the travels and what he managed to achieve. However, he regrets his cigarette smoking habits which he says had taken a huge physical and financial toll on him, making it impossible to enjoy his grandchildren as well as not leaving them enough money as planned. PC is fairly independent, lives in a retirement home with his wife, and has a helper who comes in during the day to clean. PC's children take turns to visit and care for him at the hospital since his wife has been in a wheel chair for the past 5 years.

Pathophysiology [Note 6]

[Note 7] COPD is a progressive respiratory disorder largely caused by smoking and characterized by partially reversible airflow obstruction, systemic manifestations and increasing frequency and severity of exacerbations (Global Initiative for Chronic Obstructive Lung Disease [GOLD], 2007). Chronic bronchitis and emphysema are the two most common underlying processes, usually with an overlap (GOLD, 2007). PC's diagnosis isolates emphysema. The cardinal symptoms of COPD are dyspnea, shortness of breath, cough and limitations in activity (Lewis, Heitkemper, Dirksen, O'Brien, & Bucher, 2010), with dyspnea being the most disabling symptom (Bailey, Barlett, & Beatty, 2005). These symptoms which are insidious in the onset become progressively worse, leading to an increased use of maintenance medications as well as frequent cause of medical visit. This, O'Donnell, Hernanadez, and Kaplan (2008) refer to as AECOPD and PC, who exhibited a worsened form of the above listed symptoms, is said to be at this end-stage of the disease process.

[Note 8] The normal anatomy of the lung performs the duty of oxygen and carbon dioxide exchange to and from the body via tiny sacs called the alveoli. In a COPD patient, as per GOLD (2007), inspired irritants such as smoking increase mucous production, the size and number of mucous glands in the airway, causing loss of ciliated epithelium. The mucous, which is thicker and stickier than normal, impairs ciliary function, **thereby decreasing** clearance and stimulating cough (Lewis et al., 2010). The build up traps a great number of microorganisms including the normal flora in the lungs, **activating** an infection which **accounts for** febrile symptoms and purulence of sputum (Lewis et al., 2010). **This stimulates** an inflammatory response, **causing** vasodilatation, congestion and mucosal edema (Lewis et al., 2010). The aforementioned processes **cause** narrowing of the airway lumen **resulting** in diminished airflow in and out of the lungs, especially during expiration, **increasing** the patient's work of breathing and **accounting for** expiratory wheezing. Progressive injury to the bronchioles from irritants **increases** susceptibility to infections, **leading to** scarring and stenosis, **which eventually causes** loss of elastic lung fibres and alveolar tissues (Lewis et al., 2010). According to Lynes (2010), **this reduces** the surface area of alveolar exchange, **resulting** in impaired gas exchange **and causing** sudden demand for oxygen **which leads to** shortness of breath, rapid and shallow respirations in COPD patients. COPD patients **also experience** bronchospasm **relating to** degranulation of substances from mast cells and basophils **when exposed** to irritants, allergens and air pollutants (Lewis et al., 2010). **This adds to the already increased** airway resistance, **resulting in further** increased work of breathing and impaired gas exchange.

[Note 9] PC's presenting symptoms of shortness of breath, prolonged expiratory wheezing, shortness of breath, cough with purulent sputum production and increased temperature were likely as a result from airway infection, inflammation and excess mucous build up **related to COPD**. [Note 10] PC, who was diagnosed with COPD in 1999, has been in and out of hospitals because of acute exacerbations and his presenting symptoms which led to this current hospitalization are **consistent with AECOPD**. [Note 11] Chest x-ray **suggested** chronic interstitial lung disease. His biochemistry and complete blood count lab work **indicated** an oxygen/carbon dioxide imbalance. Increased urea plasma was **suggestive of** protein catabolism; increased neutrophils and monocytes were suggestive of an infection process and inflammation mechanism; increased red blood cells count **indicated** polycythemia; and decreased MCH **suggested** low amount of oxygen-carrying haemoglobin inside the red blood cell. All these abnormal lab results ruled out other diseases and confirmed the onset of AECOPD.[Note 12] The debilitating effects of COPD on other parts of the body (Kelly, 2011) [Note 13] were not exclusive in PC's case. Decreased oxygen levels and systemic inflammation associated with COPD led to PC developing Congestive Heart failure (Sin & Man, 2003) with its related complications such as edema. PC also has weight loss due to his hypermetabolic state which requires increased energy for breathing (Schols, 2000). Lewis et al. (2010) attribute PC's muscle wasting to his episodes of dyspnea related to obstructed airways. PC, therefore, requires both acute and chronic management of his medical condition.

Pharmacotherapeutic interventions [Note 14]

[Note 15] To alleviate PC's breathlessness and other respiratory symptoms, both pharmacological and non-pharmacological interventions were adopted.

Prednisone oral glucocorticoid

Indication of use: Prednisone was prescribed to PC to relieve him of his severe and acute symptoms related to his immune response and inflammation in his airways, which was not relieved from the use of his standing medications (PRN).

[Note 16] *Mechanism of action:* Prednisone has different anti-inflammatory effects. It **acts to inhibit** the synthesis and release of inflammatory mediators such as leukotrines, histamine and prostaglandins, **thereby decreasing swelling** in PC's airways and **making in and out flow of air easier**. It **also decreases infiltration** and activity of inflammatory cells like eosinophils and leukocytes. **Hence, further damage** from release of lysosomal enzymes in PC's airway **will be averted. Lastly, it acts by decreasing** edema in PC's airway mucosa **secondary to a decrease in** vascular permeability **resulting in ease** of breathing (Lehne, 2004).

Actual or potential interactions of medications: Prednisone can increase urinary loss of potassium, thereby inducing hypokalemia. Therefore, in combination with loop direutics, a potassium depleting drug that PC is on to increase urine production, it will enhance potassium wasting effects, hence putting PC at risk of hypokalemia.

Actual or potential side effects: The short term side effects of Prednisone are nausea, diarrhea, cramps, hypertension, edema, psychologic disturbances, glucose intolerance and insomnia. Long term effects are adrenal insufficiency, osteoporosis, increased risk of infection, glaucoma, cataracts, body fat redistribution and dermatologic effects. The intensity of these effects increases with dosage size and intensity of use (Lehne, 2004).

Monitoring needs: Long term use suppresses the adrenal ability to make glucocorticoids; therefore, dosage has to be increased when stress occurs. There is the need to monitor serum potassium and advocate for supplements if needed (Lehne, 2004). Due to increased risk of infection in the use of Prednisone, PC will be informed about early signs of infection (e.g., fever, sore throat), and instructed to notify his family physician if these occur (Lehne, 2004). PC will also be educated about the signs and symptoms of fluid retention (weight gain, swelling of the lower extremities) and instructed to notify his physician if these develop.

Non-pharmacological interventions: [Note 17] As a nursing student, I was very much interested in the non-pharmacological management of PC's symptoms as there is increased **evidence that such interventions optimize** patients' functional status, quality of life, experience of dyspnea, exercise endurance, and psychosocial functioning (Lacasse, Goldstein, Lasserson, & Martin, 2006). I encouraged and assisted PC to ambulate in the hallways as and when he could tolerate **to improve** his dyspnea, **prevent** peripheral muscle wasting and overall muscle performance (Lewis et al., 2010). I also encouraged PC to engage in pursed lip breathing **to help prolong** his exhalation **and prevent** bronchiolar collapse and air trapping **which improved** his dyspnea (Lewis et al., 2010). I positioned him in high fowlers **to open** his airways **and reduce** his oxygen needs. Lastly, I facilitated the use of huff coughing **to help** PC conserve energy, **reduce** fatigue and **facilitate** removal of secretions (Lewis et al., 2010).

Future needs and follow up [Note 18]

Considering PC's frequent exacerbations with hypoxemia at rest, I would advocate for portable ambulatory oxygen equipment for him as he moves around to reduce his distress and anxiety associated with dyspnea (Brenes, 2003). PC would need the services of a physiotherapist in the first three months after discharge so as to get his mobility back to his baseline and an OT to provide him with any assistive devices he might need to help with his activities of daily living. PC cannot do as much for himself as before, so I would advocate for a caregiver to come in every day to assist him. Lastly, PC will need the services of a dietitian to manage his weight loss issues.

To control his chronic symptoms, PC would be educated on the proper administration of inhaler drugs to ensure that a good percentage is delivered to his lungs to maximize his airway patency, and should wash his mouth after every inhalation to minimize the onset of candidiasis in his mouth (Lehne, 2004). PC will also be instructed to administer bronchodilator inhalers first to dilate airways before using corticosteroid inhalers, and wait at least a minute in-between puffs to ensure efficacy (Lehne, 2004). PC will be encouraged to walk 5 to 10 minutes per day with gradual increases to improve his activity and endurance level, and to use inhaled beta-adrenergic if SOB onset is unrelieved after 5 minutes, and follow up with his family physician after a few hours of being unsuccessful. He will also be advised to have smaller, more frequent meals in a high calorie diet which is low in sodium to ensure that he gets the energy he needs for breathing, prevent bloating, and also manage his fluid retention all of which contribute to difficulties in breathing. He will also be advised to receive an annual influenza vaccination and pneumococcal vaccine (O'Donnell et al., 2008) and since he has stopped smoking, he should avoid any environmental or occupational irritants. PC will be told not to use any medications when asymptomatic (Lehne, 2004).

[Note 19] In conclusion, this paper looked at the pathophysiology of PC's diagnosis of AECOPD, explored both pharmacological and non-pharmacological interventions used to relieve his acute symptoms and future needs and education he requires to manage his chronic condition. [Note 20] Although his symptoms were relieved, the progressive, degenerative and debilitating nature of his condition will continue to have psychological consequences and effects on him, his family and carers (Guthrie, Hill, & Muers, 2001). Strict adherence and compliance with medications and regimen will decrease the risk of exacerbations, prevent acceleration of disease progression and promote his comfort and participation in care (O'Donnell et al., 2008), as well as initiate discussion of end of life issues to ensure necessary supports are in place.

Notes on sample paper 3

1   The title briefly but clearly describes the paper's topic (COPD) and its focus (pathophysiology and pharmacotherapeutics).
2   This introduction received 5/5 marks. The criteria were:
    o   brief introduction of case, roadmap of what will be discussed, how it will be discussed;
    o   clarity;
    o   conciseness.
3   The first paragraph gives a brief introduction to the case and the focal presentation of COPD.
4   The second paragraph provides a clear outline – the roadmap – of the three sections of the paper:
    a) pathophysiology;
    b) pharmacotherapy;
    c) nursing implications.
5   This important section describes all the relevant details of the patient that form the background for the presenting illness. Demographic information is important for three reasons:
    o   because an individual's personal history and circumstances often provide clues to medical diagnosis;
    o   because nursing and midwifery treat the whole person, not just the symptoms they are experiencing; and
    o   because these factors may contribute to or impede recovery.

Thus, the section includes dimensions of both medical history and life history, such as age, gender, developmental stage, language, family and social supports, socioeconomic status, and cultural/religious influences. It also includes the history of the focal presentation. It should include all the information that is relevant to the focal presentation (but no extra or 'interesting' information) and also say why it is relevant.

6   This assignment did not include a differential diagnosis section. If it had, the structure would be similar to the pharmacotherapy section in this sample paper. In a differential diagnosis, bullets or subheadings are used to list the possible

diagnoses, moving from most to least probable. Under each diagnosis, subsections describe:

- o the evidence for, based on the patient's presenting symptoms and the research literature;
- o the evidence against, based on the same criteria;
- o the tests that could be performed to confirm or refute the diagnosis, from most important test to least;
- o a conclusion as to which tests should be ordered in this case.

A patho paper that includes a differential diagnosis section may ask for a discussion of pharmacotherapy for only the most likely diagnosis, or for all the possibilities.

This section of the sample paper received 23/25 marks. The criteria were:

- o explanation of pathophysiological process;
- o clarification of any chronic issues and how they are related to the focal presentation;
- o genetic or lifestyle factor involvement, if relevant;
- o clinical manifestations supportive of focal presentation;
- o diagnostic tests that support diagnosis.

Describing a pathophysiological process involves a type of writing called 'process analysis'. A process is a series of connected actions, each developing from the one before it, and leading to some result. We describe a process in chronological order, like a story, but can interrupt the story/account to discuss its relevance. For complicated processes, we distinguish the main stages and the steps within each one.

7 The first paragraph gives definitions relevant to the focal presentation, moving from most general (COPD) to most specific (AECOPD).

8 The words that are bolded in this paragraph show the causal sequence of events in the COPD process.

9 The first part of the paragraph links the patient's presenting symptoms to the COPD process described in the last paragraph.

10 The verbs and verb phrases bolded in this paragraph function to relate the symptoms and test results to the focal presentation.

11 The next part of the paragraph describes the tests used to confirm the diagnosis.

12 Notice that the diagnosis is reached both by ruling out other diseases and by confirming the AECOPD.

13 Notice that the argument here and throughout the paper is carefully evidence-based.

14 Only one sample drug therapy of the four that the paper describes is included here. All followed the same format. This section received 24/25 marks. The criteria were:

- o   related drugs, mechanism of action, reason for use;
- o   drugs' relation to clinical manifestations;
- o   any interactions or clinical considerations;
- o   relation to pathophysiological process.

For each possible drug therapy, this section should describe:

- o   the mechanism of action and reason for use;
- o   relation of the drug to the clinical manifestations;
- o   any interactions or clinical considerations;
- o   relation to pathophysiological process.

15 The section begins with a brief statement that summarizes the content and organization of the section.

16 The bolded words in this therapy section, like the ones in the patho section, act as links to the COPD process, but in this case they are words suggesting improvements in the process.

17 In this section, bolded words show the positive effects of nursing interventions on the COPD patho process.

18 The monitoring and follow-up section should explain monitoring needs, acute and chronic management, potential side-effects, and discharge planning (such as education, management, ongoing follow-up). This section received 21/25 marks. The criteria were:
- o   discuss monitoring needs and why;
- o   acute and chronic management and rationale for same;
- o   potential side effects or clinical considerations;
- o   discharge planning, if necessary (education, management, ongoing follow-up).

19 The conclusion received 4/5 marks. The criteria were:
- o   brief summary;
- o   review of patho and pharm connection;
- o   clarity, conciseness.

The final paragraph provides a succinct summary of the paper. The first sentence of the concluding paragraph repeats the outline of the paper's structure given in the paper's introduction.

20 The paragraph continues to the end with an overall picture of PC's follow-up.

INDEX